Superfoods

How to Make Them Work For You

Julie Neville

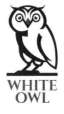

WHITE
OWL

First published in Great Britain in 2017 by
Pen & Sword White Owl
an imprint of
Pen & Sword Books Ltd
47 Church Street
Barnsley
South Yorkshire
S70 2AS

ISBN 978 1 52671 733 7

Typeset in Meta by
Mac Style Ltd, Bridlington, East Yorkshire
Printed and bound in Malta by Gutenberg Press Ltd.

Pen & Sword Books Limited incorporates the imprints of Atlas,
Archaeology, Aviation, Discovery, Family History, Fiction, History, Maritime,
Military, Military Classics, Politics, Select, Transport, True Crime, Air World,
Frontline Publishing, Leo Cooper, Remember When, Seaforth Publishing,
The Praetorian Press, Wharncliffe Local History, Wharncliffe Transport,
Wharncliffe True Crime and White Owl.

For a complete list of Pen & Sword titles please contact
PEN & SWORD BOOKS LIMITED
47 Church Street, Barnsley, South Yorkshire, S70 2AS, England
E-mail: enquiries@pen-and-sword.co.uk
Website: www.pen-and-sword.co.uk

Superfoods

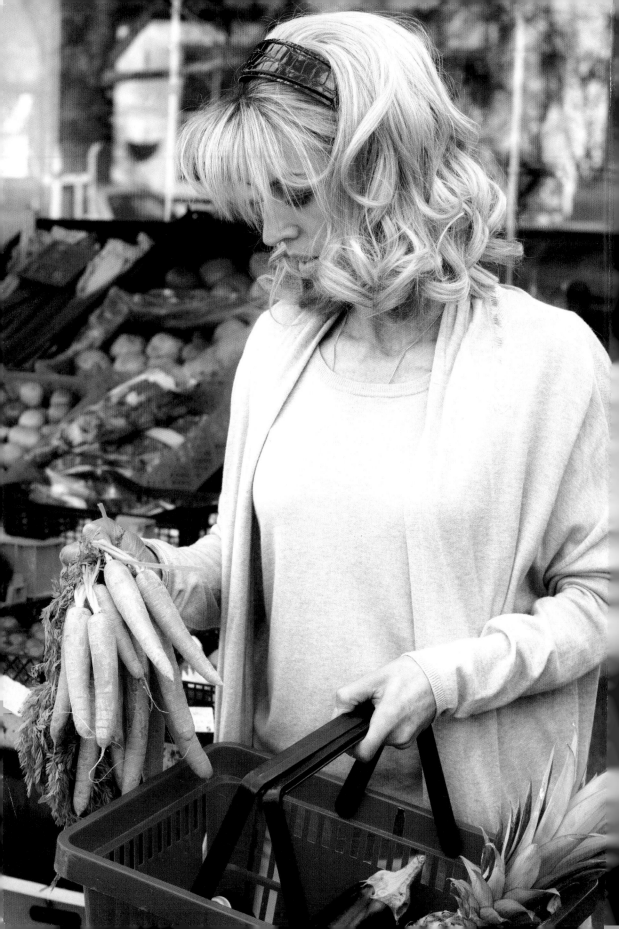

Contents

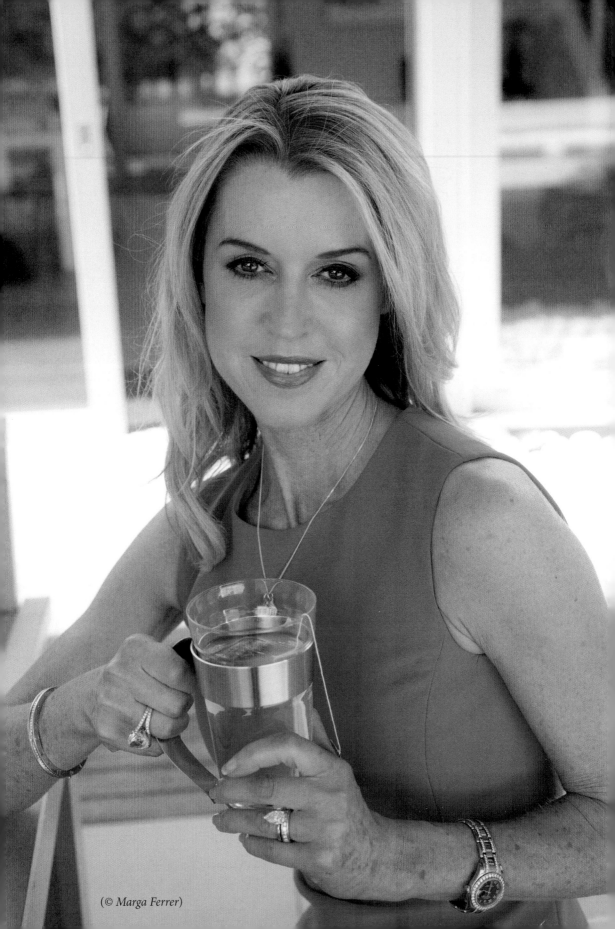

Superfoods

By Julie Neville

According to the Oxford Dictionary, a superfood is 'a nutrient rich food that is considered to be especially beneficial for health and wellbeing.' The Macmillan Dictionary states a superfood is 'a food that is considered to be very good for your health and may even help some medical conditions.' For me, a superfood is simply a food that is nutrient dense so bursting with vitamins and minerals. An added benefit is that these powerful foods can be energizing, anti-ageing, calming, anti-inflammatory, healing to both body and mind and may prevent disease.

In recent years, the term 'superfood' has become the buzzword in terms of food and health, and every single day the media is filled with reports of the latest ultra-healthy food. While this is on the whole a positive trend, the huge influx of information can be both overwhelming and confusing.

I have followed the superfood phenomenon with great interest over the past decade, and I have been desperate to discover whether these superfoods were actually 'super' after all. Could adding these potent items to our diet on a more regular basis really have a huge impact on our health? And after 10 years of investigation, I can happily conclude that the answer is YES! As a result of eating superfoods regularly my family has more energy, more powerful immune systems, clearer skin, stronger nails and hair, balanced hormones, fewer illnesses, and a more rapid recovery from injuries. In addition, my family has been cured of a wide range of health conditions, and I honestly believe that eating superfoods might have saved my life during a health crisis some years ago. Now on the rare occasion that anyone in my family starts to show signs and symptoms of any illness, my first stop is never the chemist but my cupboard of what I like to call my 'natural cures', and they never let me down! I would even go as far as to say that I healed my body with these special foods.

A common misconception is that superfoods are weird and wonderful potions that most have never heard of, and are even less likely to be able to pronounce. Well, hopefully in this book I can dispel that myth and prove that superfoods are often simple foods that the majority of people will have sitting in their fridge or cupboards. I also hope to demonstrate how easy they are to incorporate into a daily diet for the whole family and how delicious they are. There are a limited number of foods we can eat in a day, and with

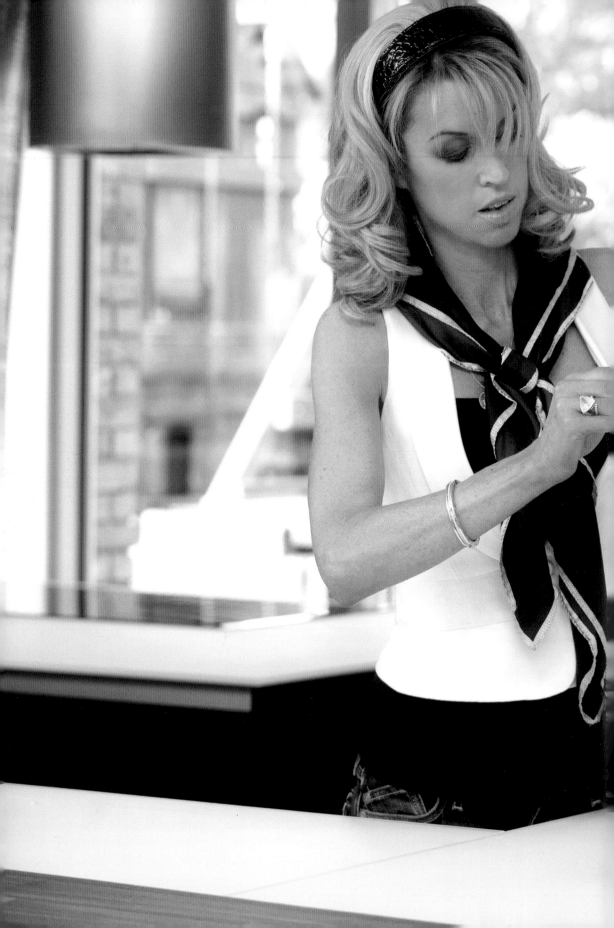

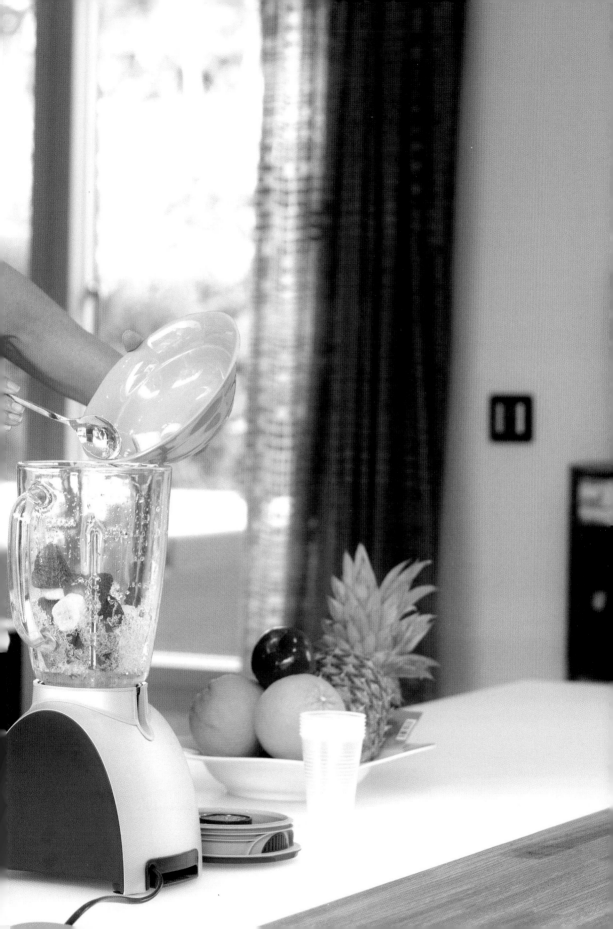

this book I aim to help you to choose the ones that carry the greatest amount of nutrients and will be most beneficial to the body. I have also added in a few helpful hints to give your everyday foods a powerful super charge.

In order to simplify things further, I have categorized the foods into various sections. I am certain you will be surprised to read of the health benefits of items that you probably walk past in the supermarket every single week – maybe next time they will make it into the trolley!

Before we start to work our way through what is certainly a fantastic list of superfoods, I think it is important to talk briefly about the importance of healthy food choices. I am going to reveal in depth the benefits of a wide range of foods, but I also feel it is worthwhile to just highlight briefly the effects of poor diet choices.

Make no mistake – eating poorly for even a short period of time has negative consequences. In 2009 an American study on rats proved that eating a fatty meal had an immediate negative impact on brain function. Eating a restricted diet or skipping meals also had similar effects, including poor memory and poor concentration levels.

Bad diet choices also lead to fatigue – you have probably all experienced that mid-afternoon slump at some point. Low muscle strength, physical weakness, low endurance and weak coordination are all common in people who make poor nutritional choices. Consuming greasy and fatty foods, eating too fast, overeating, drinking too much caffeine or alcohol can lead to heartburn, indigestion, nausea, bloating and acid reflux. A poor quality diet undoubtedly leads to low quality sleep and that in itself can lead to a whole host of other problems. Long term poor quality sleep is debilitating to both the mind and body.

The chemicals in our brain that promote positive moods rely on food and nutrients for proper function. A lack of such nutrients can not only lead to low moods and depression but also tension, anger and irritability. Poor dietary choices can result in weight gain, and there are a number of reasons for this. Usually, junk food is high in fat and calories but they also lead to further cravings and overeating. So to re-cap briefly, just a few of the short-term effects of poor diet choices include:

- **Reduced brain function**
- **Fatigue**
- **Dull or acne prone skin**
- **Poor muscle strength**
- **Diminished coordination**
- **Low endurance**
- **Physical weakness**
- **Heartburn**
- **Indigestion**
- **Bloating**
- **Acid Reflux**
- **Poor quality sleep**
- **Depression**
- **Anger**
- **Irritability**
- **Tension**
- **Weight gain & obesity**

That may seem like a shocking list but these are just the short- term effects of poor diet choices – the long-term consequences make even more shocking reading, and include:

- **Tooth decay**
- **High blood pressure**
- **High cholesterol**
- **Heart disease**
- **Stroke**
- **Type 2 diabetes**

- **Osteoporosis**
- **Cancer**
- **Liver failure**
- **Kidney stones**
- **REDUCTION IN LIFESPAN!!!!!!**

That ultimately sums it up for me – long-term poor diet choices reduce the length of your life!

I am certain that after that final statement, you will need little encouragement to make healthier choices. And the changes you may need to make really are quite simple and affordable.

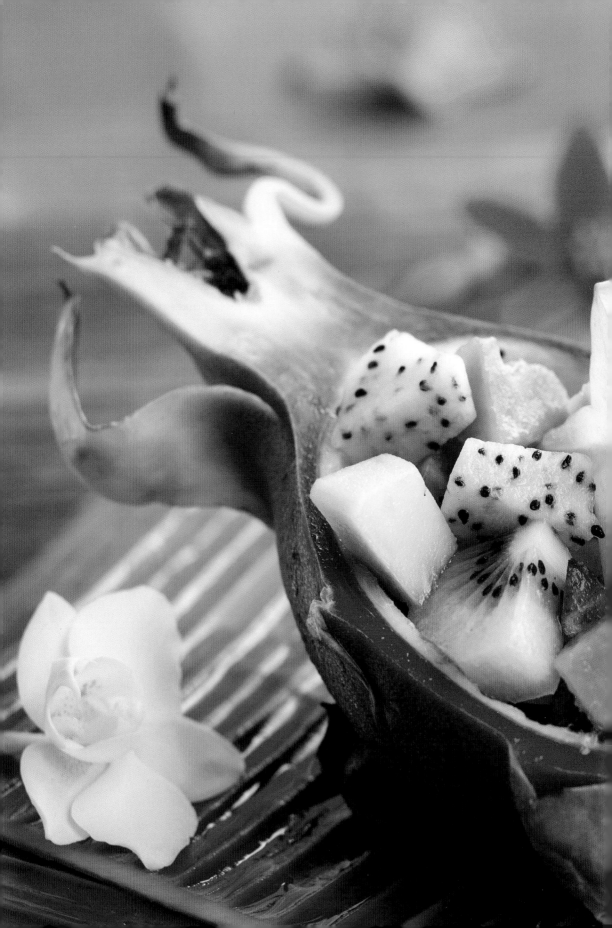

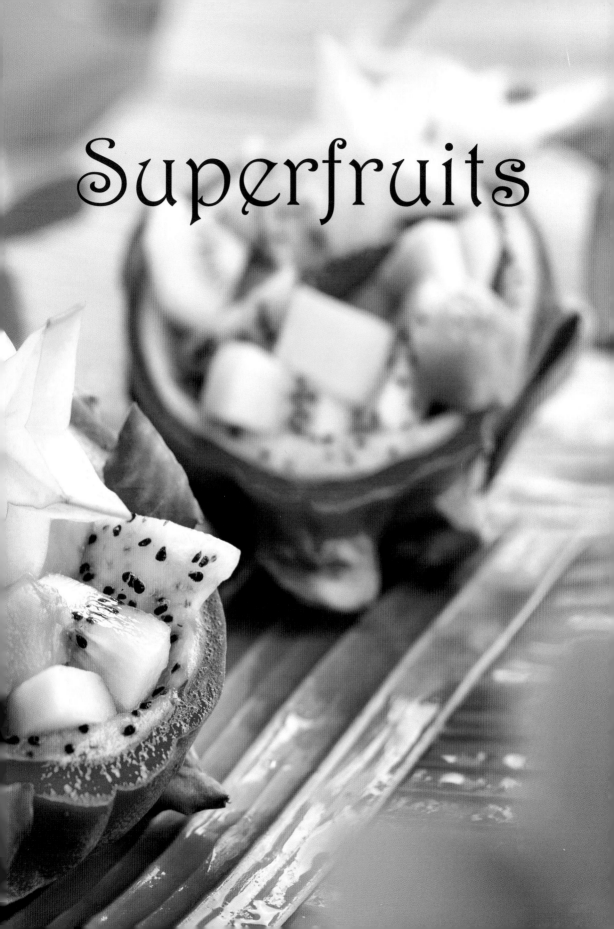

Superfruits

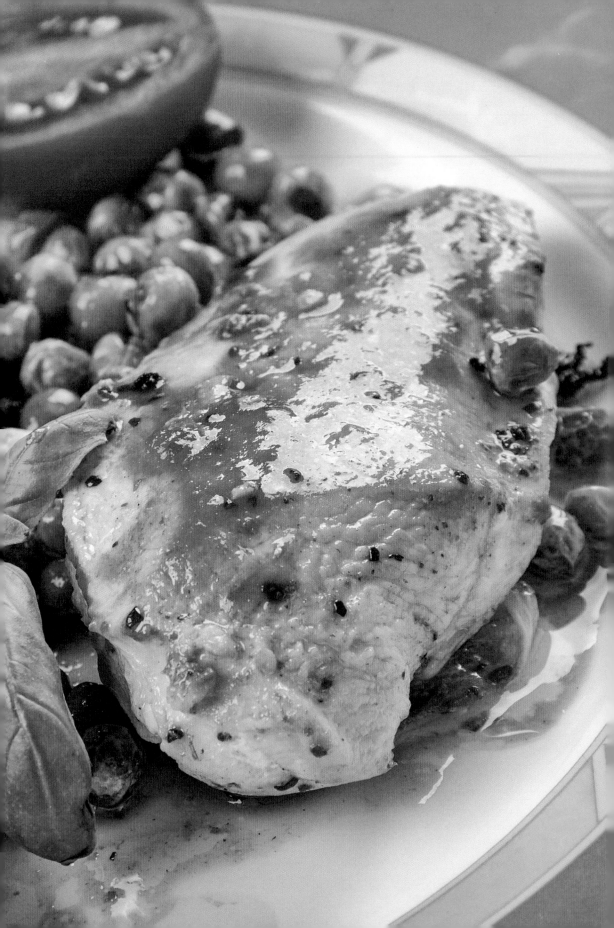

Believe it or not, despite their reputation as being healthy, not all fruits are classed as superfruits. To earn this title, they have to be rich in antioxidants, fibre, vitamins and minerals. So like most other foods, not all fruits are equally healthy. Also, it is best to eat fruit whole and fresh, not pre-prepared. So which ones should we be stocking up on?

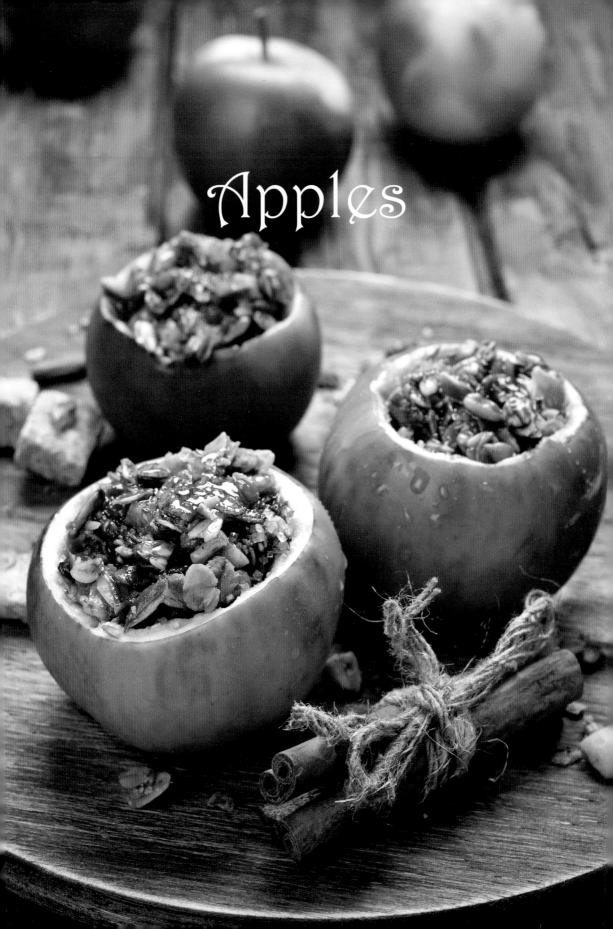

Apples

Low Fat Vegan Apple Banana Bread

Ingredients

1 apple peeled and sliced
2 ripe bananas
Just under 2 cups of whole wheat flour
½ a cup of apple sauce

1 tablespoon of baking soda
1 teaspoon of cinnamon
1 teaspoon of salt
1 teaspoon chopped walnuts

Preheat the oven to 180°C and lightly grease a loaf tin.

In a bowl, mash the bananas then add all the other ingredients except the walnuts and mix well.

Pour into the loaf tin and sprinkle with the chopped walnuts.

Bake for approximately 45 minutes until a toothpick placed in the centre of the loaf comes out dry.

Leave to cool in the pan for 15 minutes.

This is delicious for breakfast smothered in peanut butter or even for a healthy dessert!

So the famous saying of 'an apple a day keeps the doctor away,' really is true. Apples are rich in fibre and antioxidants (our disease fighting compounds). The soluble fibre in apples binds with fat in the intestines, leading to lower cholesterol levels. This soluble fibre also prevents sugar swings. In fact, a recent study by Harvard School of Public Health revealed that people who eat more wholefruits like apples have a lower risk of developing Type 2 diabetes. Never peel your apples before eating them as the skin contains quercetin which is a powerful antioxidant that has antihistamine and anti-inflammatory properties, which may protect you from heart disease and allergic reactions.

Uses – There is no need for any guidance on how to use this famous fruit, quite simply eat it as nature provided it – although dessert doesn't always need to be naughty and apples make an easy and delicious pudding. Baked apples with a gooey, oat topping are a favourite in our house.

Avocados

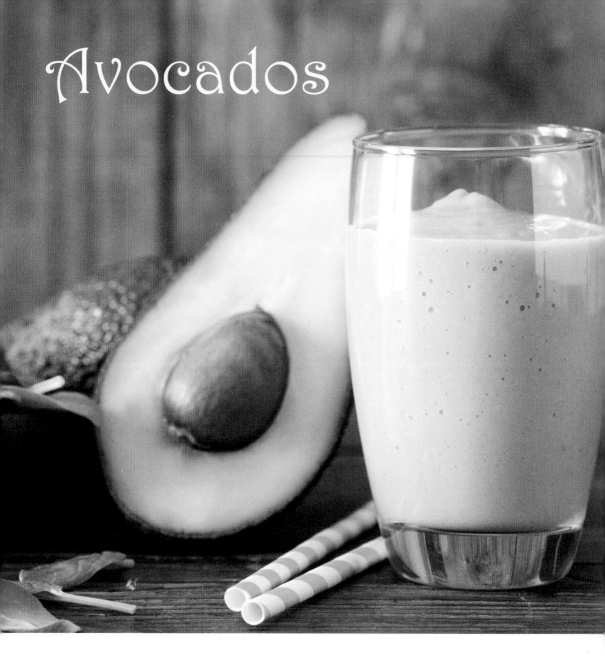

Avocados are by far one of my favourite fruits (yes they really are a fruit) and I eat two of them every single day, usually blended into my superfood green smoothies in the morning. They are packed with monounsaturated fats and fatty acids (healthy fats) which help to lower bad cholesterol levels (LDL) and raise good levels. Avocados are considered to be one of the healthiest foods on the planet as they contain over 25 essential nutrients, including vitamins A, B, E and C as well as copper, iron, phosphorus, magnesium and potassium. Their B6 and folic acid content help to regulate homocysteine – high levels of which are associated with an increased risk of heart disease.

They are rich in a compound known as beta sitosterol which has been shown to be effective in lowering blood cholesterol levels. They are an excellent source of potassium

The Neville Super Smoothie

Ingredients

2 apples

1 orange

½ a cucumber

2 sticks of celery

6 large carrots peeled

2 handfuls broccoli florets

3-4 inch piece of ginger (I actually add much more than this but normal people prefer a little less than my rations of ginger)

2 handfuls of spinach

2 handfuls of kale

2 handfuls of watercress (If easier you can just add one whole mixed bag of salad leaves)

2 avocados peeled and with the stone removed

Using a juicer, juice all the ingredients except the avocados.

Place the avocados into a blender or Nutribullet then add the juice.

Prior to blending, I also add protein powder as well as other superfood powders which I choose daily depending on my mood or nutritional requirements.

Blend until thick, smooth and creamy then enjoy!

which helps to control blood pressure levels and they have superb anti-inflammatory properties. Their lutein content helps to promote eye health whilst their high folate content can prevent birth defects and reduce the risk of strokes. Their powerful antioxidants fight free radicals within the body, slow down ageing, boost the immune system and promote a healthy nervous system.

Uses – Avocado oil is often added to cosmetics as it is so nourishing to the skin; mashed avocado makes an excellent face mask and can also be effective in treating eczema and psoriasis. As for their culinary merits, they are incredibly versatile, and can be added to salads, used to make guacamole or creamy, healthy chocolate desserts, added to sandwiches or wraps, and as a key ingredient in a green smoothie. I have one every day as they are so delicious and energizing.

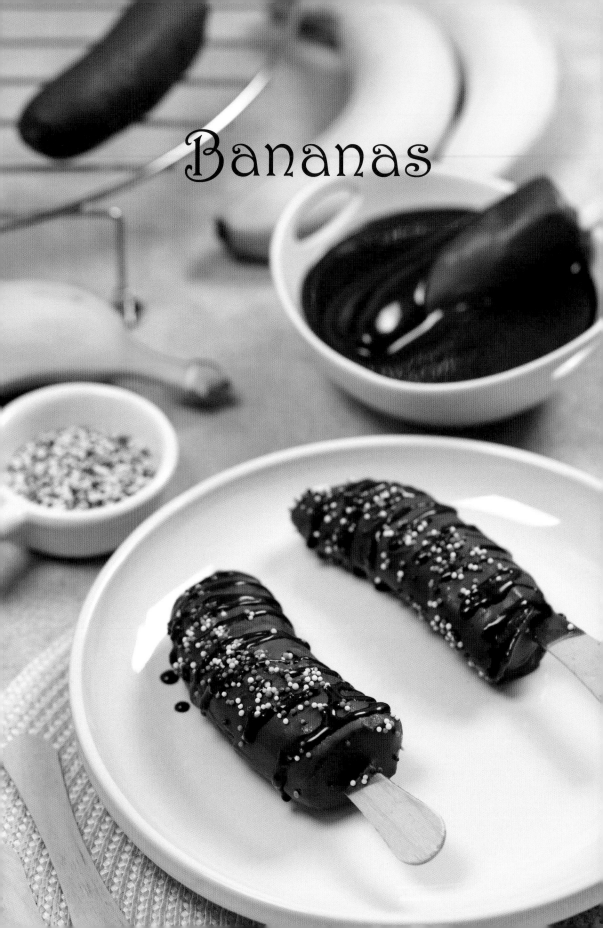

Bananas

Quick and Easy Grilled Bananas

If you have never had grilled or barbecued bananas then you really are missing out. They are so quick and simple to make and are always a crowd-pleaser.

Simply cut the ends off the ripened bananas and leave in their skins. Grill or barbecue them on a medium heat for around 10 to 15 minutes. The skins will turn black and start to crack.

Open the skin down the middle to expose the warm grilled, bananas and serve with honey and cinnamon or syrup or a little sugar. My daughter also loves to squirt cream onto hers.

Bananas are one of the most popular fruits on earth. They are a rich source of resistant starch – a healthy carb that helps to fill you up, and to boost the metabolism. Bananas are bursting with potassium (which most people do not get enough of) and which helps to lower blood pressure. They are also rich in fibre, antioxidants and nutrients. Each banana contains almost no fat and on average, just over a hundred calories. They can help in the balance of blood sugar levels and digestion. Bananas are also often referred to as 'athletes' food' due to their easily digested carbs and high mineral content. They are an excellent fuel for endurance exercise and may also prevent muscle cramps and soreness. They really are one of the most convenient snacks around but also easy to incorporate into baking. My children love to freeze them then dip them in melted chocolate to freeze once more, before making a delicious yet healthy treat!

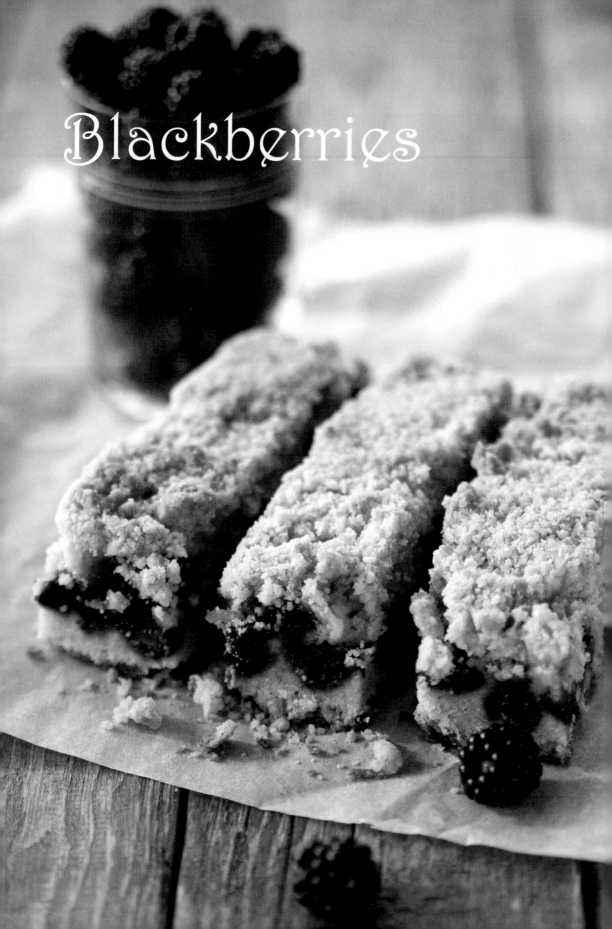

Blackberries

Blackberry Crumble

Ingredients

1½ cups of all-purpose flour
¾ cup of light brown sugar
½ cup of cold unsalted butter cut
   into small pieces
2¾ lbs fresh blackberries

Two tablespoons of instant tapioca
¾ cup of granulated sugar
1 tablespoon grated orange zest
¼ cup of orange juice

Preheat the oven to 180°C then place the butter, brown sugar and flour into a food processor and pulse until combined.

In a separate bowl, place the blackberries, granulated sugar, tapioca, orange zest and juice and mix together before pouring into a baking dish.

Pour the flour mixture over the top. Bake in the oven for around 45 minutes until the topping is golden and the fruit mixture is bubbling.

Cool for around 15 minutes before serving with custard.

These tart, deep purple berries always bring back wonderful childhood memories of walking with my basket to collect berries from the blackberry bush, before rushing home with my stash to my mother and begging her to let us bake with them. Their dark purple colour indicates that these little berries have a super high concentration of antioxidants. In fact, they are in the top ten for antioxidant power for fruits, according to the ORAC table which measures the levels of antioxidant per calorie in all foods. Not only that, they are extremely low in calories with only 62 calories per cup yet super high in fibre with 7.6gms per cup which is more than a bowl of bran flakes.

There is strong evidence to suggest that their vitamin content may help to prevent heart disease and age related decline. A 2009 study published in the medical journal *Nutritional Neuroscience* stated that blackberry intake may have a positive impact on cognitive and motor skills which often decline with age. Blackberries may also improve oral health as they contain gallic acid, rutin and ellagic, compounds which have antiviral and antibacterial properties. Gargle blackberry juice to treat sore throats, mouth ulcers and inflamed gums.

Uses – Don't think that blackberries are only good for jams, they are wonderful in crumbles and pies, with pancakes and scones, blackberry compote with yoghurt is delicious and frozen blackberries blended to make a sorbet or frozen dessert is simply divine!

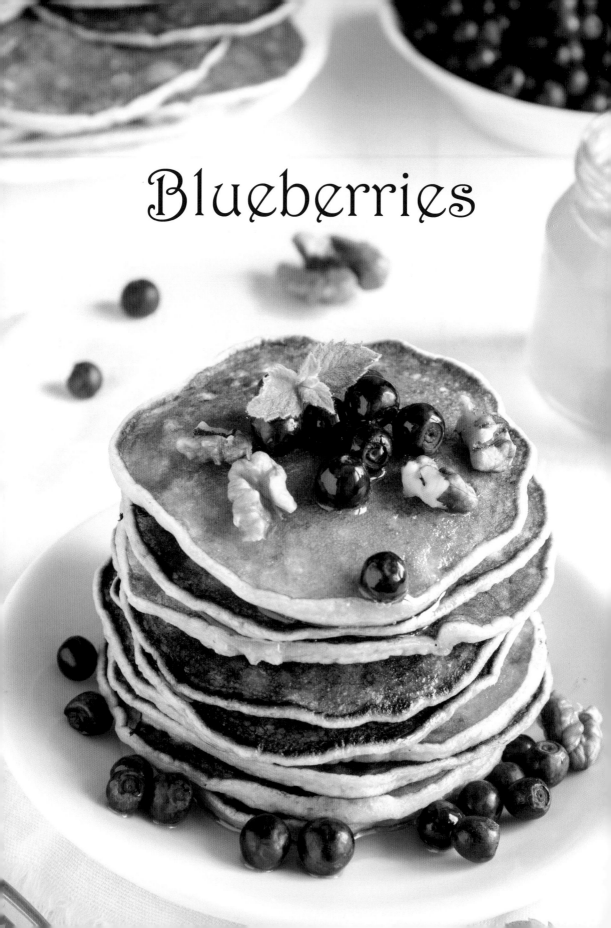

Blueberries

Chunky Blueberry Sauce

Ingredients

2 cups of fresh or frozen
   blueberries

½ a cup of honey

1 teaspoon of freshly grated lemon
zest

2 tablespoon lemon juice

Place all the ingredients into a saucepan and bring to the boil stirring continuously.

Reduce the heat and simmer for around 15 minutes until the sauce has thickened, stirring occasionally.

Leave to cool for around 10 minutes, then serve whilst still warm. This sauce will keep in the fridge for one week or in the freezer for up to one month.

I love this sauce as it makes a fantastic addition to yogurts, fruits, pancakes, muffins and ice cream and it is simply delicious.

Blueberries have received a lot of media coverage in recent years. Sweet, nutritious and low in calories, blueberries are rich in fibre, vitamin K, vitamin C and manganese. They are thought to contain the highest concentration of antioxidants of all commonly consumed fruits and vegetables. Antioxidants protect our bodies from damage by free radicals which are unstable molecules that can interfere with cell structures, leading to ageing and diseases. Their main antioxidant compound are flavonoids, and many studies have proven that consuming blueberries and blueberry juice regularly can have a significant impact on preventing DNA damage and there is also evidence to show that eating blueberries can help to prevent heart attacks.

However, blueberries seem to be most recognized for their benefits to brain function and delaying age-related decline. My children adore blueberry pancakes, and my husband and I love blueberries added to our porridge for an extra boost to start the day.

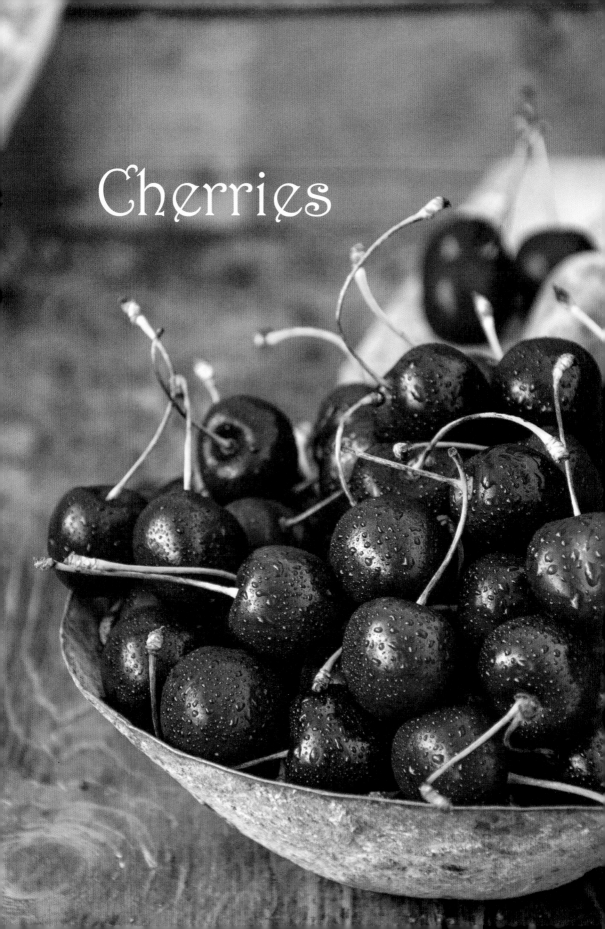

Cherries

Cherry Pistachio chocolate bark

Ingredients

200g high quality, dark chocolate
¾ of a cup of unsalted shelled
  pistachios

½ a cup of chopped dried cherries
Handful of dried cherries and
  pistachios for topping

Place the chocolate into a bowl and place it on top of a pan of boiling water, stirring until all the chocolate has melted.

Add the cherries and pistachios and stir well until all the nuts and fruits are coated.

Pour the mixture onto a baking sheet and spread well and then sprinkle with chopped pistachios and cherries before placing in the freezer to set for one hour. Remove and break into pieces to serve.

Cherries, for me, really are the heroes of superfruits as they have so many health benefits and only contain 87 calories per cup. They are packed with antioxidants known as anthocyanins which aid in the reduction of heart disease and cancer. They are also an excellent source of beta carotene, a pigment that is converted into vitamin A in the body. Cranberries contain 19 times more beta carotene than strawberries and are also rich in vitamins E, C, magnesium, potassium, iron, folate and fibre.

Often referred to as 'brain food' they help to prevent memory loss. Cherries are one of the few foods that contain melatonin which helps to regulate heart rhythms and sleep cycles. A glass of cherry juice before bed will most definitely be more effective than counting sheep! Cherries have proven to be particularly effective in reducing inflammation and have had great success in treating arthritis and gout. This powerful anti-inflammatory effect has made cherries a popular choice for athletes keen to reduce muscle pain and soreness and to improve post-training recovery times. A bowl of cherries in our house never lasts long, but they are also great for jams, fruit compotes, and desserts.

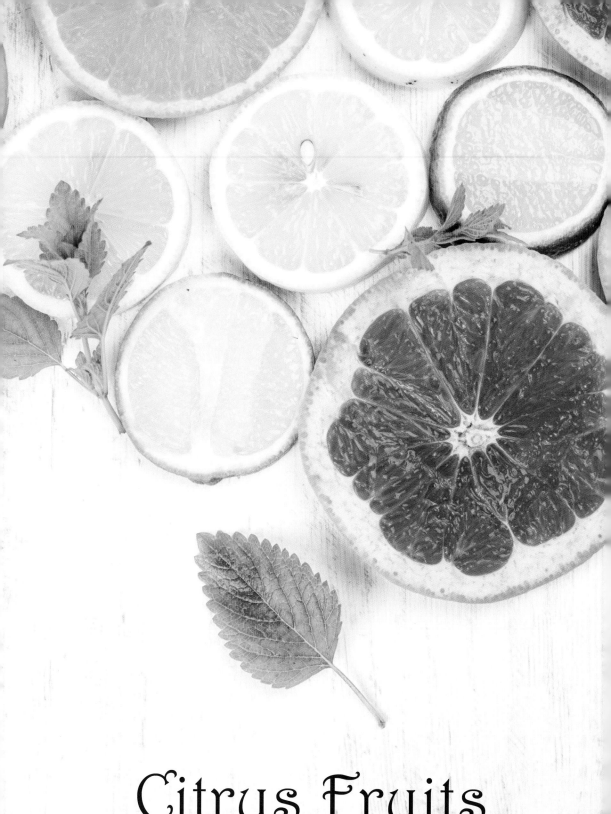

Citrus Fruits

Summer Citrus Salad

Ingredients

1 large orange
1 large grapefruit
2 small fennel bulbs, sliced finely
¼ cup extra virgin olive oil

¼ cup fresh basil leaves
¼ cup toasted chopped walnuts
Salt and pepper to taste

Peel both the grapefruit and orange, and then release each segment from its membrane by carefully slicing along the membrane until the segment comes out easily. Do this over a jug so that any juice that is released is caught.

Place all segments into a bowl with the sliced fennel. In a blender or food processor, blend together the oil, basil leaves and two to three tablespoons of juice from the jug.

Season with salt and pepper then pour over the citrus fruits and fennel and toss in the chopped walnuts. Mix until all ingredients are coated well and serve.

Citrus fruits include oranges, lemons, limes, grapefruit, tangerines and pomelos. They are rich in vitamin C which helps the body to absorb iron by binding it to the digestive track. Vitamin C is also used for the synthesis of collagen which helps wounds to heal and to hold blood vessels, ligaments, tendons and bones together. They are rich in flavonoids which for a quick reminder, can neutralize free radicals and may protect against heart disease. It is thought that they improve blood flow through the arteries by reducing their ability to form blood clots and build up plaque on the artery walls. Finally, they are a good source of folate and B vitamins.

We currently live in Valencia which is famous for its oranges. Everyone makes freshly squeezed Valencia orange juice daily and so this has become a healthy habit of ours. On the school run in the morning, we pass the fruit trucks collecting the oranges and then the next morning we juice them. However, citrus fruits also go well with salads and many other dishes, so experiment and enjoy!

Interesting Fact – Did you know that squirting lemon juice on freshly cut fruits, avocado or guacamole prevents them going from going brown and helps them to last longer?

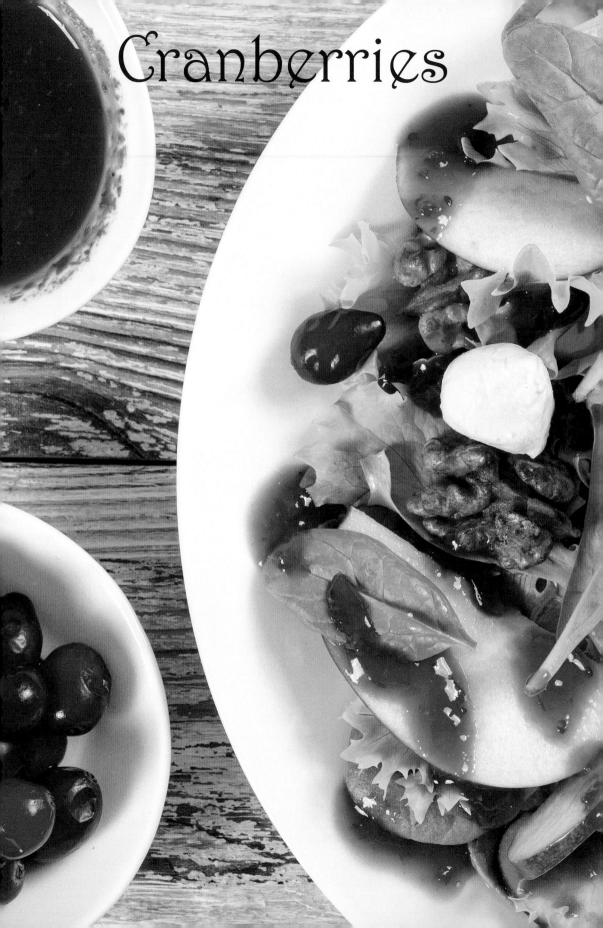

Cranberries

Cranberry, Walnut and Gorgonzola Salad

Ingredients

A large bowl of salad greens of your choice

½ cup walnuts

½ cup cranberries dried

½ cup gorgonzola cheese crumbled

1 tablespoon olive oil

1 tablespoon raspberry vinaigrette

1 tablespoon white wine vinegar

The walnuts can be candied in this recipe if want to make it sweeter. Start off by adding them to a pan with quarter of a cup of sugar.

Stir continuously over a medium heat until all the sugar dissolves into a liquid and all the walnuts are coated.

Remove from the heat and pour the walnuts onto a baking sheet and leave to cool while you assemble the rest of the salad.

Add the cranberries and gorgonzola to the salad leaves.

In a jug, mix together the vinaigrette, olive oil and white wine vinegar and then pour over the salad leaves.

Toss all the ingredients until mixed and coated well. Once the walnuts have cooled and set, pour into the salad and toss again.

These tart little berries have long been praised for their qualities in preventing urinary tract infections. Drinking cranberry juice may inhibit bacteria from sticking to the walls of the bladder thus preventing UTIs. Also according to a new study from Rutgers University, in New Jersey, cranberries can increase the effectiveness of chemotherapy drugs used to treat ovarian cancer and may slow the growth of cancer cells. Another study found that people who drank a glass of cranberry juice daily, raised their HDL (good cholesterol) by ten per cent.

Uses – For me the easiest way to consume cranberries is through the juice which is widely available and delicious although I have also found that dried cranberries make a fantastic substitute for raisins in baking recipes.

Interesting Fact – Want to know if your cranberry is fresh? Then simply drop it on the floor. Fresh cranberries bounce and if they don't bounce then they are rotten!

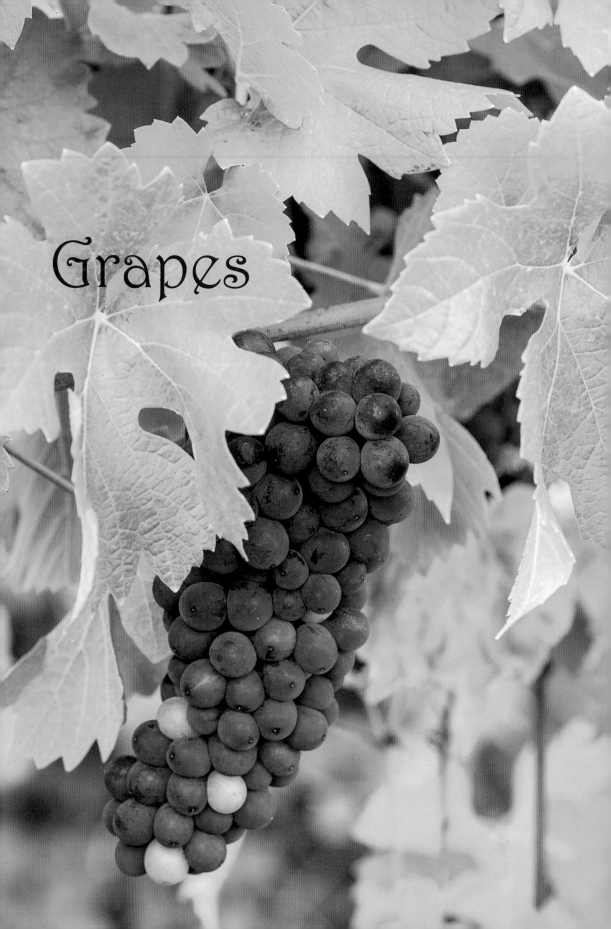

Grapes

Grape Jelly

Ingredients

2 packets of unflavoured gelatin

2lbs red seedless grapes (around
   five and a half cups)

Additional grapes to decorate

½ cup of sugar

2 to 3 cups sour cream

2 tablespoons honey

Put half a cup of water into a bowl and sprinkle over the gelatin and allow it to soften.

Place the grapes, sugar and one cup of water into a medium saucepan. Bring to the boil then reduce the heat and simmer pressing the grapes occasionally to break and loosen the skins – this can be done with a spoon or even a potato masher, and should take between 10 and 15 minutes.

Add the gelatin to the pan with the grapes, and stir until dissolved completely. Strain the mixture through a fine mesh sieve pressing to extract as much liquid as possible. You may need to add a little water as you press.

Divide the liquid between four serving glasses and place in the fridge to set for a minimum of two hours.

Stir together the sour cream and honey and spoon onto the top of the now set jelly. Garnish with sliced grapes.

Grapes gain their superfruit status due to their high content of the powerful antioxidant resveratrol which promotes a healthy heart. Compounds found in grapeseed extract have also shown positive effects at slowing Alzheimer's disease. One cup of grapes (approximately 32 grapes) contains just over a hundred calories and virtually no fat. An excellent source of vitamins C, A, potassium and folate, the high water content in grapes makes then an excellent choice for hydrating. However, the Environmental Working Group include grapes in the fruits with the highest pesticide content so always buy organic and wash well before eating.

Uses – Grapes fit perfectly when sliced in half and added to fruit cocktails or salads but we love to pop them in the freezer for a delicious healthy treat in the summer too. And grape pops always seem to be popular with our children.

Fact – The malic acid in grapes naturally breaks down the stains and discolouring on teeth!

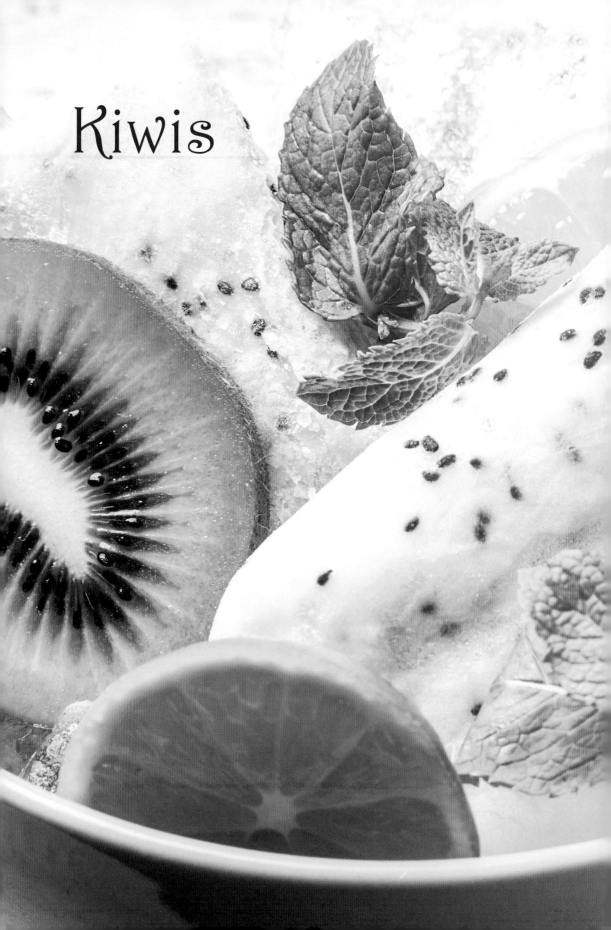

Kiwis

Tropical Kiwi Lollipops

Ingredients

1 can (14oz) coconut milk
1 chopped banana
1 cup chopped kiwi

Sliced kiwi
¼ pineapple chopped

Pour the coconut milk into a blender adding the pineapple and banana.

Blend until smooth then stir in the chopped kiwi.

Place the whole slices of kiwi along the sides of the moulds before pouring the mixture in.

Freeze for a minimum of eight hours or overnight.

I always think of kiwis as being like a treasure chest – not particularly attractive on the outside with their brown, hairy skin but when you cut them open, their vibrant green or golden centre is revealed. Since ancient times, kiwis have been thought of as a health tonic in China, and were given to women after childbirth. I am always drawn to any fruit salad with bright green kiwis and not just because they are super tasty, but kiwis also have a host of health benefits; one of the most well-known being their success in treating the symptoms of irritable bowel syndrome or constipation. A study undertaken by a group of scientists showed that participants who ate two green kiwis daily for four weeks reported significant improvements in their IBS and bowel problem symptoms.

The International Kiwi Organization also did a study that proved that people eating kiwi fruit daily showed higher levels of DNA repair compared to those who didn't eat them. Another study was undertaken by a kiwi company which showed that eating two kiwis before bedtime significantly increased total sleep time and sleep efficiency by 13.4 per cent and 5.41 per cent respectively, and concluded that kiwis may improve sleep onset, duration and efficiency. In addition, they are rich in fibre, contain several vitamins and minerals as well as slow digesting carbohydrates. They also have multiple health benefits, as kiwis also help to balance the acid and alkaline levels in the body which is extremely important for overall health. They have anti-ageing benefits and at only 46 calories per average fruit, this makes them a fantastic choice.

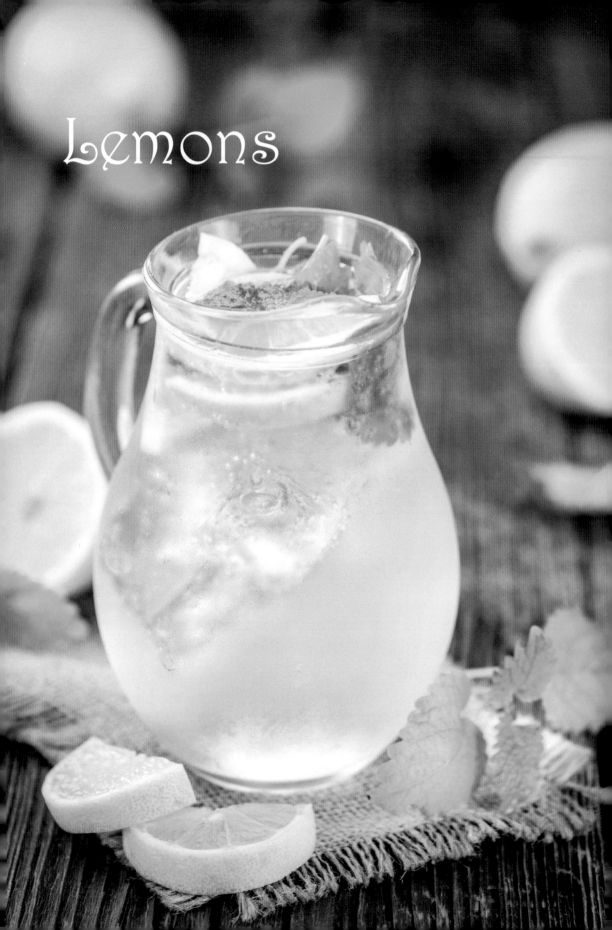

Lemons

Chicken Piccata

Ingredients

4 skinless, boneless chicken breasts
½ cup white wine
½ cup freshly squeezed lemon juice
¼ cup water
2 tablespoons olive oil
2 tablespoons capers

3 tablespoons cold, unsalted butter
2 tablespoons fresh, chopped
  parsley
A little flour for dredging
Salt and pepper to taste

Place the chicken between the cling film and pound with a rolling pin until around quarter of an inch in thickness.

Season the chicken with salt and pepper then dredge in the flour shaking off any excess.

Heat the olive oil in a pan and add the chicken. Cook over a medium heat until golden and cooked through then remove from the pan and keep warm.

Add the capers to the pan and cook for around 30 seconds before adding the white wine.

Cook for a further two minutes until the wine has reduced a little before adding the lemon juice, water and butter.

Cook for two to three minutes until the sauce thickens before adding the parsley.

Return the chicken to the pan for a few minutes more, and then serve with the sauce spooned over the top.

Although obviously a citrus fruit, I thought it was important to single lemons out as they have been used for generations to treat a wide range of ailments, including throat infections, constipation, fever, burns, respiratory disorders and high blood pressure just to name a few. Also used to clean the skin and hair, they are thought to be a blood purifier, an excellent stomach cleanser and immune booster. Lemon juice has been shown to prevent the occurrence of kidney stones and drinking lemon juice and olive oil is known to get rid of gallstones (albeit not the tastiest thing you will ever drink).

Lemon is a natural antiseptic, it is effective on skin problems, burns and stings; and the well- known old remedy of lemon juice, honey and hot water will not only bring a glow to your skin but will also relieve cold and flu symptoms. Lemon is also calming to both the body and mind and is often used in the treatment of anxiety and depression. It has effectively been used to treat arthritis symptoms and I can now confidently say it is an excellent mosquito repellent too. Lemon in water with ice is a truly refreshing drink and excellent on waking to cleanse the system.

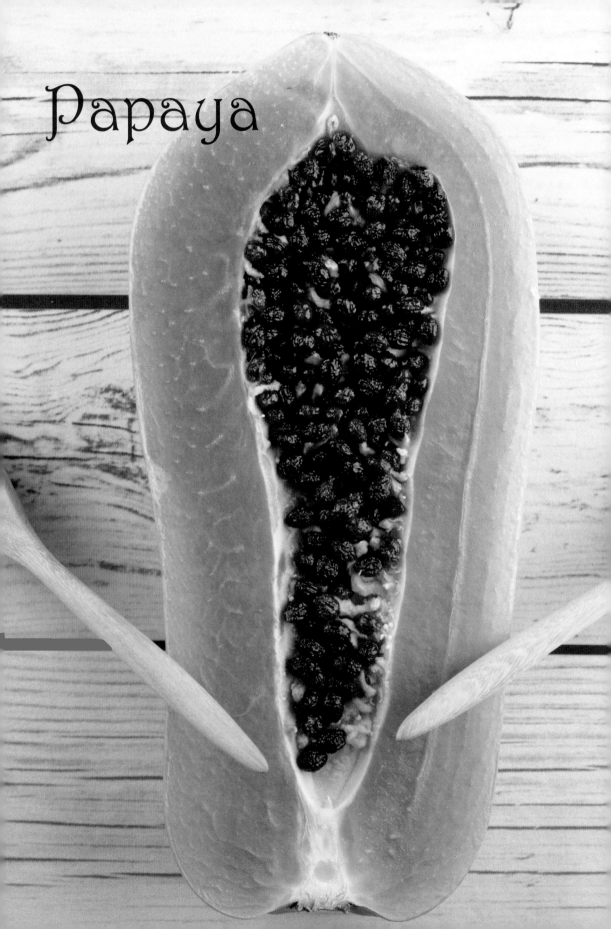

Papaya

Papaya Boats

Ingredients

2 papayas cut in half length way and seeded

1 cup of fresh strawberries chopped

2 tablespoons honey

1 cup of natural yoghurt – Greek yoghurt works well as it is thicker and creamier

¼ cup raisins

Mix all the ingredients together then load into the papaya halves – slice a couple more strawberries to decorate the top.

This bright, exotic fruit is both sweet and refreshing but did you know that it is rich in fibre, vitamin C and antioxidants and may even lower cholesterol? Its fibre content promotes a feeling of fullness and can prevent cravings and so aids weight loss. Just one papaya provides 200 per cent of our daily vitamin C requirement giving us a fantastic immune boost. This fruit's low sugar content and glycaemic content makes it an excellent source of nutrition for diabetics. Rich in vitamin A and beta carotene which promotes healthy eyes, it also has anti-inflammatory properties which help to reduce the symptoms of arthritis. The enzyme papain is fantastic for digestive health and can also regulate and ease the flow of menstrual cycles. Rich in anti-ageing properties, it boosts hair and can reduce stress – making it an-all round super power fruit.

Uses – Papaya works well in smoothies, is delicious stuffed with yoghurt and berries, and in fruit salads. It makes a fantastic salsa but it also suits poultry and fish really well.

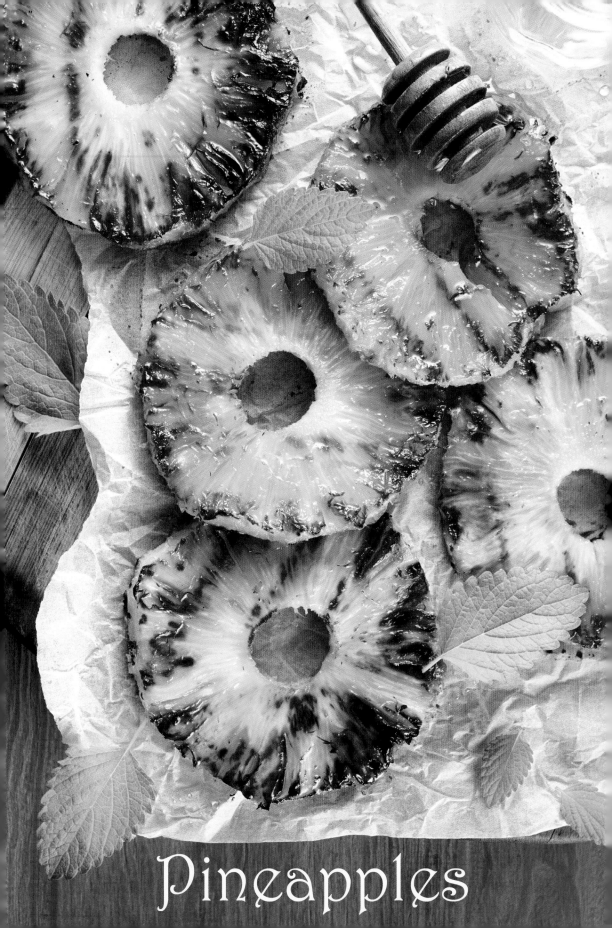

Pineapples

Pineapple Bran Muffins

Ingredients

1 cup of raisins
1 cup of wheat bran
1 level cup of all-purpose flour
1 teaspoon baking powder
½ teaspoon of baking soda
½ a cup of plain yoghurt

½ cup of molasses
¼ cup of dark brown sugar
½ cup of melted butter
1 large egg
1 can (20oz) pineapple drained and
   chopped

Preheat the oven to 180°C and place bun cases in two muffin trays – 18 in total.

Cover the raisins with boiling water and leave for ten minutes to soften, drain then puree in a blender or food processor until smooth.

In a bowl, combine the bran, flours, baking soda and baking powder.

In a separate bowl, stir together the yoghurt, sugar, molasses, butter, egg and raisin puree. Add the dry ingredients and stir to combine. Carefully fold in the pineapple chunks before spooning the mixture into the muffin cases.

Bake for around 25 minutes in the oven until a toothpick inserted into the centre of a muffin comes out clean and dry.

I ADORE pineapples! Now they are found in every grocery store and most homes. Used for centuries to treat digestive problems and inflammation, their fibre and water content may aid constipation. Being rich in antioxidants as well as copper, zinc and folate makes pineapples a fertility boosting food. As they have a high vitamin C content they can boost collagen, improving skin health and the immune system. Pineapples' combination of vitamin C and bromelain has shown positive effects in its treatment of colds and flu symptoms. The enzymes in pineapple have also been shown to reduce inflammation in the nasal cavity and break up excessive mucus in the respiratory system. One cup of pineapple contains three-quarters of our daily recommended intake of manganese which is vital for our bodies to build healthy bones and connective tissues. Manganese also assists in energy productions and the B vitamins in pineapples make them a fantastic stress buster.

Uses – Delicious as a juice or grilled on a barbeque, sweet and sour chicken is always popular but also try blending them with ginger to make a nutritious smoothie, adding to salads or baking in loaves and muffins, skewered with red onions and fish or in curries.

Interesting Fact – Christopher Columbus brought pineapples back to Europe after one of his trips to South America. At the time, they were considered lavish and exotic and were served only at banquets.

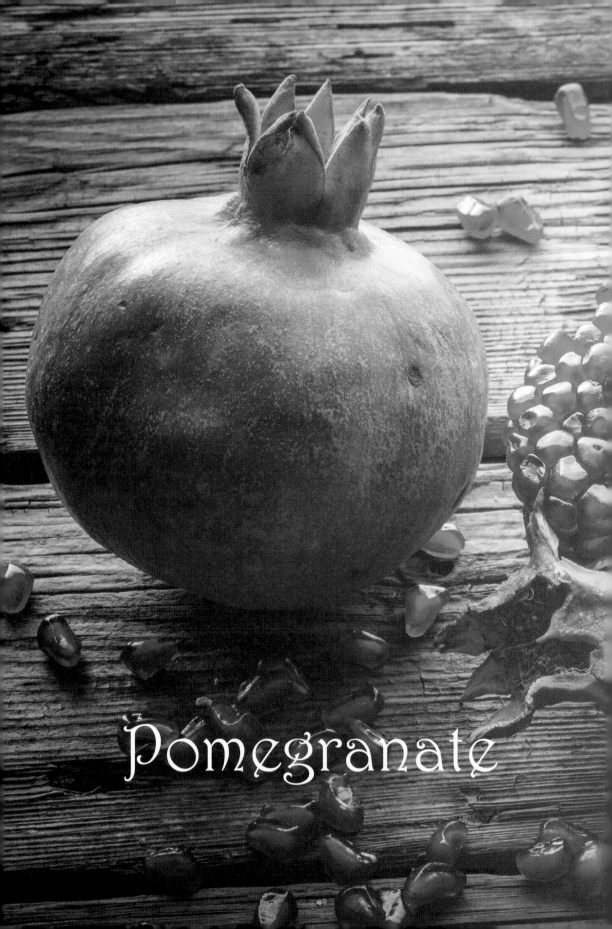

Pomegranate

Sweet Potatoes with Coconut, Pomegranate and Lime

Ingredients

4 sweet potatoes
½ cup of coconut milk
¼ cup of toasted coconut flakes
  (unsweetened)

1 tablespoon chopped cilantro
1 cup pomegranate seeds
Lime wedges
Salt

Preheat the oven to 200°C

Prick the sweet potatoes and bake then in the oven for around 45 minutes until soft on the inside.

In a bowl, mix together the pomegranate, coconut milk, coconut flakes and cilantro.

Slice open the sweet potatoes, make a well in the soft flesh within and load with the pomegranate mixture.

Sprinkle with a little sea salt and top with lime wedges.

Pomegranates have a leathery texture on the outside but inside their seeds are juicy and sweet. They too are rich in antioxidants, as well as vitamin C, with 300ml containing almost half a person's daily requirement. They have high amounts of vitamin K which helps to support bone health whilst manganese aids the formation of bone structures making it an all-round bone healthy fruit. High in phosphorus, calcium, magnesium, iron and zinc, they contain very little fat and no cholesterol, and pomegranates have been shown to increase skin cell regeneration and circulation, which slows ageing by preventing age spots, fine lines and wrinkles. They also help the body to produce more elastin and collagen and to improve dry skin making them a super beauty food too.

Pomegranate juice can act as a blood thinner, and helps to remove plaque from the arteries as well as aiding digestion and working as an extremely effective laxative in treating constipation. Its high iron content can help to raise haemoglobin levels and treat anaemia. Pomegranates can be used as a gargle for sore throats or used directly on the skin to treat haemorrhoids. I like to use pomegranates in juice form, with the seeds added to my porridge or I add them to quinoa and salad.

Tomatoes

Tomatoes are so easy to include in your diet and once you read of their multiple health benefits you will be certain never to leave them off your plate again. Their bright red colour is owed to their rich content of the antioxidant lycopene which according to the *British Journal of Nutrition* is linked to an almost 30 per cent reduction in the incidence of cardiovascular disease. They are super rich in B vitamins and also vitamins A, K and C as well as folate, potassium, iron, magnesium and chromium. They improve the function of the digestive system and the liver as well as reducing constipation and can also prevent both kidney stones and gallstones as well as reducing the risk of urinary tract infections.

Due to its vitamin K content, drinking tomato juice greatly improves the quality and texture of the hair. Tomatoes also stimulate the production of the amino acid carnitine which has shown to increase the body's fat burning capacity by over 30 per cent, making it an effective weight loss tool. They can help protect the body from eye degeneration, boost the immune system and prevent blood clots. Recent research in the journal *Harvard Health Letter* found that diets rich in tomatoes can also help to prevent strokes and even cancer.

Uses – There is no better use for them than in a delicious tomato sauce to add to pasta or vegetables or a winter warming homemade tomato soup. But if you do want to be more adventurous, then stuffed tomatoes make a fantastic starter and tomatoes roast wonderfully with aubergines.

Important tip: Although there is a loss of vitamin C when tomatoes are cooked, the beneficial phytochemicals are significantly raised during the cooking process increasing their heart healthy and cancer fighting properties.

Roasted Red Pepper and Tomato Soup

Ingredients

1 tablespoon olive oil
1 chopped onion
2 cloves garlic minced
3 red bell peppers
4 large tomatoes, peeled, seeded and chopped
2 teaspoons thyme
2 teaspoons paprika

1 large pinch of white granulated sugar
6 cups of vegetable stock
2 tablespoons butter
A pinch of cayenne pepper
1½ tablespoons flour
6 tablespoons sour cream
A dash of hot sauce, if required

Rub oil on the peppers then place under the grill for 15 minutes, turning so all the sides blacken.

Remove and place into a paper bag for a further 15 minutes. This will enable you to remove the skins, cores and seeds easily.

Core the peppers and keep one pepper aside.

Heat the olive oil over a medium heat and add the onion and garlic and cook for around five minutes until soft but not browned.

Add the tomatoes, peppers, paprika, thyme and sugar and cook for approximately 25 minutes until all the tomato juices have evaporated.

Add the stock, hot sauce (if required), and salt and pepper.

Bring to the boil then reduce the heat and simmer for around 25 minutes until all the vegetables are softened.

Strain the soup then place the solids into a blender and blend until smooth before adding back into the liquid.

In a separate large pan, melt the butter then add the flour and cook for one minute.

Slowly start to add the soup, stirring continually. Once all the soup has been added to the butter and flour, add the reserved chopped pepper and stir.

Bring back to the boil then simmer for a further ten minutes.

Ladle into bowls and topped with a tablespoon of sour cream or I like to simply swirl with olive oil.

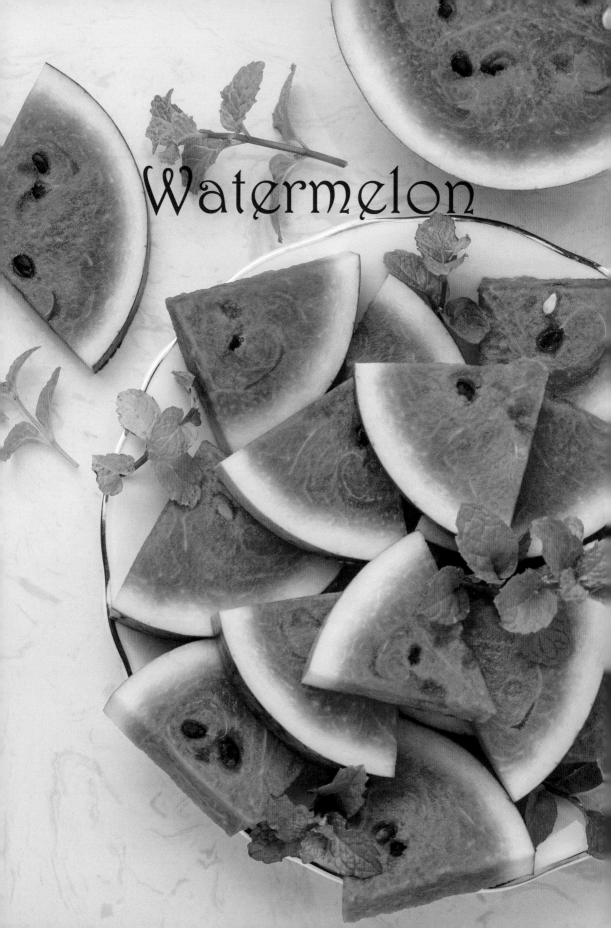

Watermelon

Melon Fruit Salad Bowl

Ingredients

2 large water melons

2 cups of cantaloupe melon balls

2 cups of water melon balls

2 cups of blackberries

2 cups of strawberries

1 cup of blueberries

1 cup raspberries

Cut the watermelons across the centre but in a zig zag design – you may want to mark the circumference prior to starting to ensure you remain in the centre all the way round.

Once in two halves, use the centre part only of the melon to make your water melon balls, hollowing out a little of the centre of the melon halves but leaving the zig zags towards the edges.

Mix together all the fruits then load back into the watermelon halves. How lovely does that look!

In season, during the summer, watermelons are a truly healing fruit. Naturally low in fat and extremely hydrating, they have a 92 per cent water content. Rich in lycopene, which is important for both cardiovascular and bone health, they help to reduce blood pressure and their potassium content helps the body to retain calcium. Watermelon contains citrulline which is an amino acid which with the help of our very clever kidneys turns into arginine which boosts circulation. When consumed, citrulline has the ability to make our fat cells create less fat thus preventing the accumulation of overall body fat, and is a natural anti-inflammatory and diuretic, which helps our liver and kidneys to remove excess waste and fluids. Watermelon has an alkaline effect on our bodies preventing illness and disease and they are also rich in vitamin C so boosting the immune system. For me, the best and only way to eat watermelon is straight from the fridge and freshly sliced!

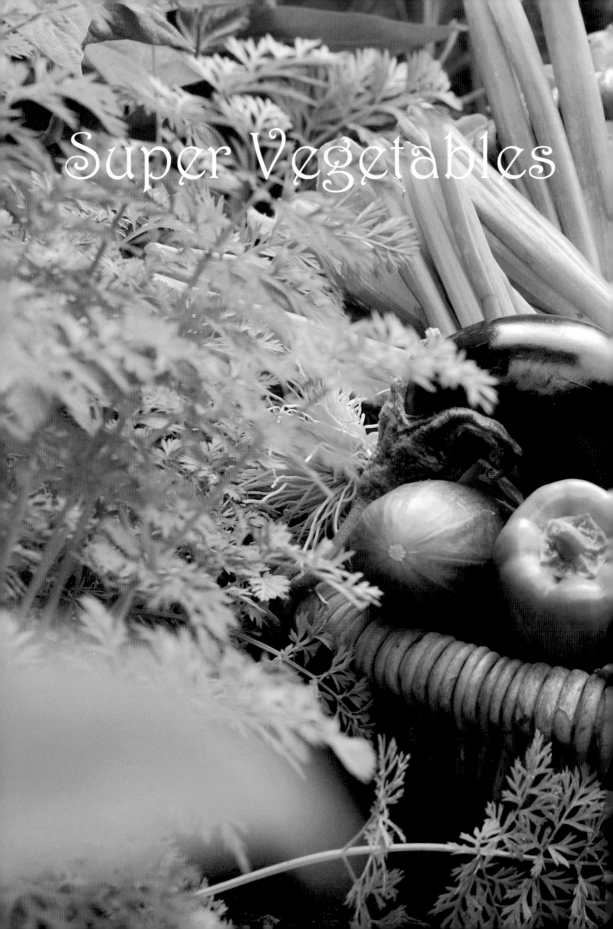

Super Vegetables

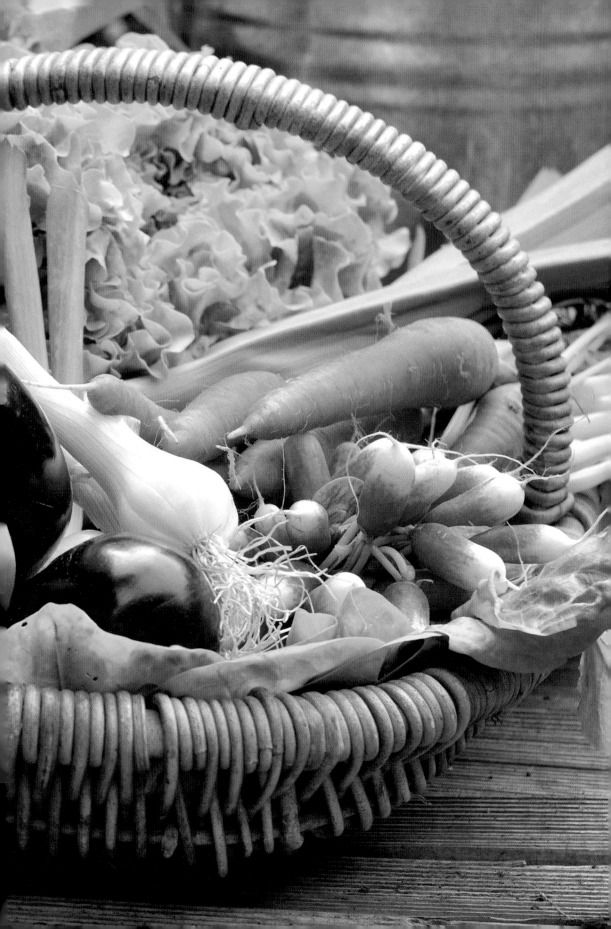

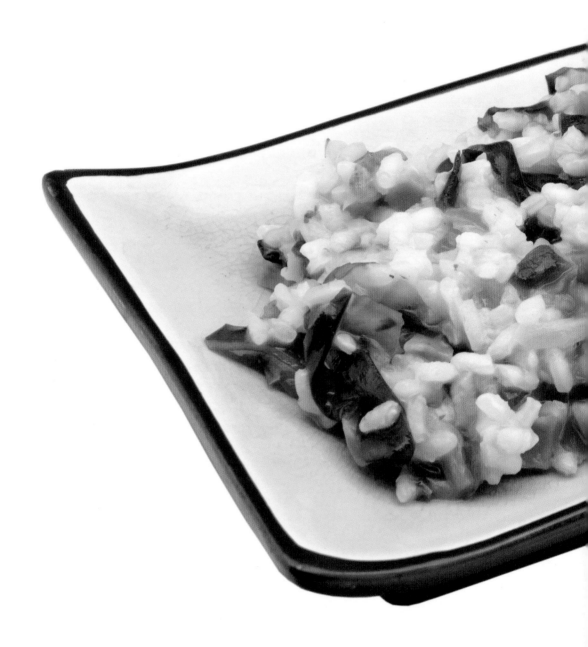

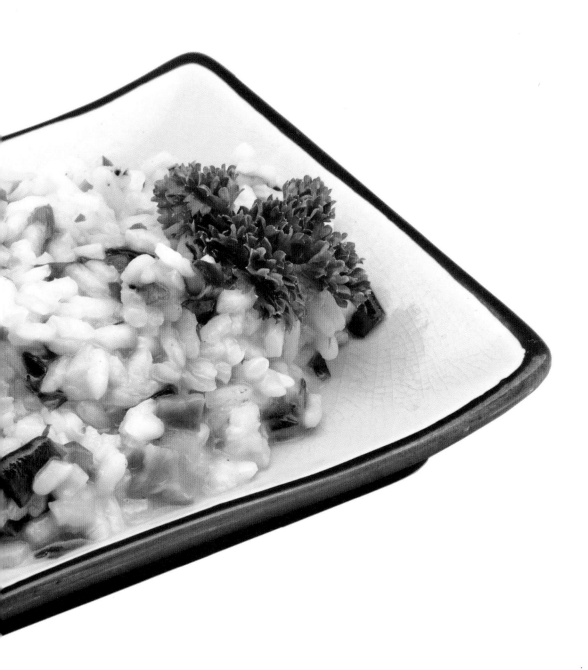

Although all vegetables are good for us, they are not all equally nutritious. So which ones should we be incorporating into our daily diets? Below I have listed what I consider to be the most potent and nutrient dense vegetables.

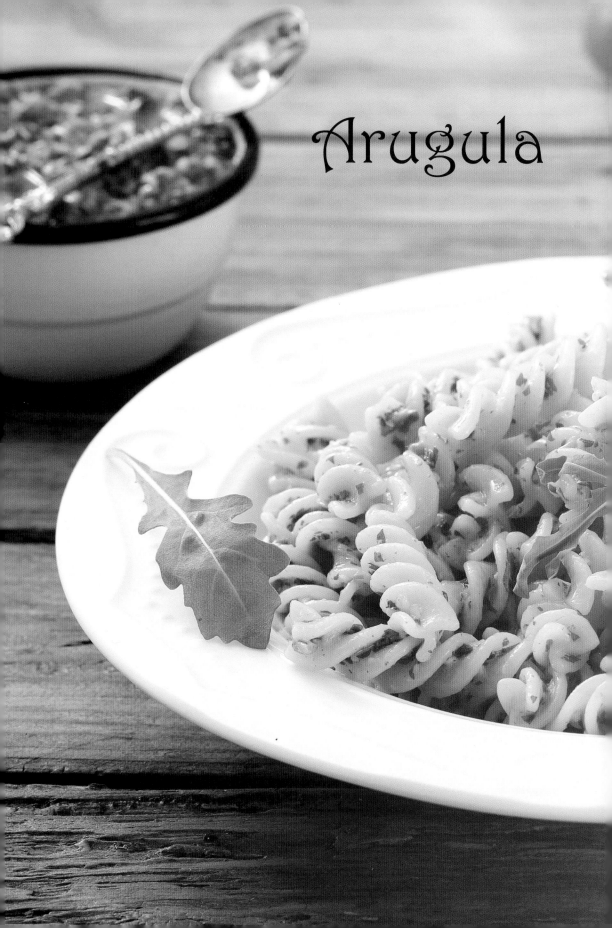

Arugula

Pasta with Arugula Pesto

Ingredients

¼ cup of chopped walnuts
3 cloves of minced garlic
2 cups of chopped arugula
¼ cup of chopped fresh basil

½ cup olive oil
1/3 cup of grated parmesan
Salt and pepper
16oz of dried pasta of choice

Combine the garlic, arugula, walnuts and basil in a food processor and blend until coarsely chopped then whilst blending, add the olive oil until smooth.

Stir in the parmesan, salt and pepper. Cook the pasta as per instructions then drain and return to the pan. Stir in the arugula pesto before serving into bowls and sprinkling with a little more parmesan and topping with basil leaves.

Although given its appearance it may not be obvious, but arugula is closely related to radishes, cabbage and cauliflower. Also commonly known as salad rocket, this peppery vegetable has a long list of healing properties. Arugula is a leafy, green plant packed with vitamins, minerals and antioxidants. It provides a fantastic defence against free radicals, cancer, premature ageing and heart disease. Another bone healthy vegetable with a high vitamin K content and a natural anti-inflammatory, arugula is a good source of vitamin C and folate, making it an excellent choice for pre-natal women and the high B vitamin content promotes metabolic health.

Uses – You have probably all eaten arugula with shaved parmesan and olive oil but it can be used for so much more. Add it to soups, sandwiches, pastas and use it to make a delicious homemade pesto!

Interesting Facts – Arugula grows to a height of between 20 to 100 cm and is recognizable by its small white flowers. Did you know that many centuries ago the Romans discovered a rather unlikely effect of this leafy green vegetable? That it acted as a powerful aphrodisiac!

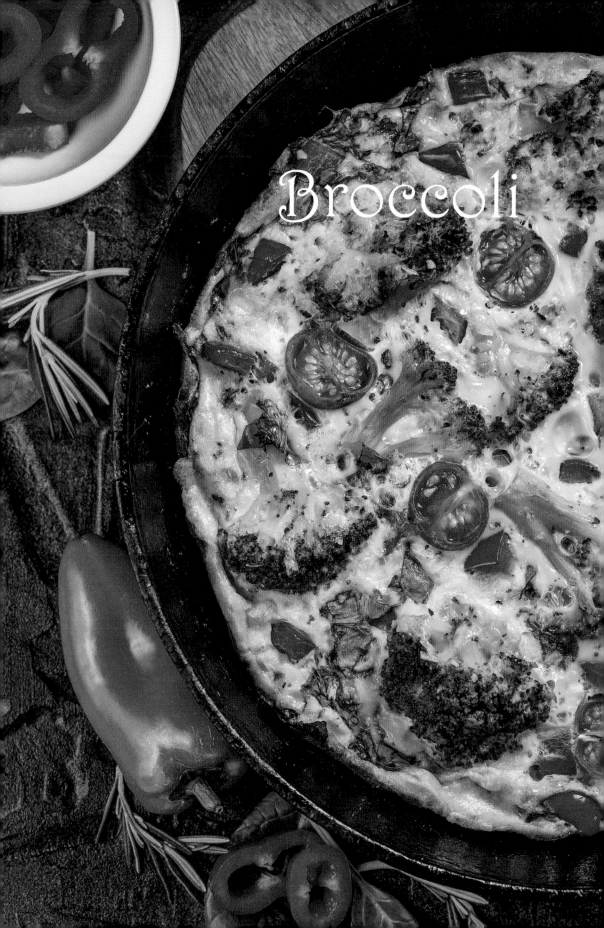

Broccoli

Broccoli Frittata

Ingredients

2 tablespoons olive oil
1 garlic glove sliced
3½ cups of broccoli florets
¼ of a red pepper diced finely

8 large eggs
½ a cup of grated parmesan cheese
Salt and pepper

Preheat the oven to 175°C, then in a large non-stick pan, heat one tablespoon of olive oil and add the garlic cooking it for only 30 seconds but on a high heat.

Add the broccoli and pepper and cook for a couple of minutes more before adding two tablespoons of water, and then, season with salt and pepper then cover.

Cook over a medium heat for a few minutes until the broccoli is tender but still crisp, and then remove from the heat and leave to cool.

In a bowl, whisk the eggs, season with salt and pepper then add the broccoli and pepper mixture.

Heat the remaining olive oil in the pan then pour the egg mixture into the pan. Cook over a low heat until set around the edges which will take around three to four minutes.

Sprinkle with the cheese then transfer to the oven and bake for a further 10 to 12 minutes until the centre of the frittata is set.

It is great served with freshly baked baguettes and a large salad.

The humble broccoli probably sits in the majority of fridges yet most people probably don't know the full extent of its nutritional benefits. A member of the cruciferous family, broccoli provides numerous nutrients for very little calories. It is rich in folate and both vitamin K and calcium, providing a boost to bone health. One cup of broccoli provides more vitamin C than we require in one day, boosting the immune system and skin health, and helping to keep wrinkles at bay. Broccoli is a good source of natural fibre, preventing constipation, promoting a healthy digestive tract and aiding the removal of toxins and waste from the body. According to the Department of Internal Medicine and Nutritional Sciences programme at the University of Kentucky, high fibre intakes are associated with significantly lower risks of developing coronary heart disease, stroke, hypertension, diabetes, obesity, high blood pressure and high cholesterol. Broccoli ranks in the top 20 of nutritious foods in the world, according to the Aggregate Nutrient Density Index.

Uses – Broccoli is really easy to incorporate into your diets and even that of your children. Try sautéed broccoli with olive oil and pepper, add to soups and smoothies, roast it, stir fry it, make soups with it and add to pasta sauces.

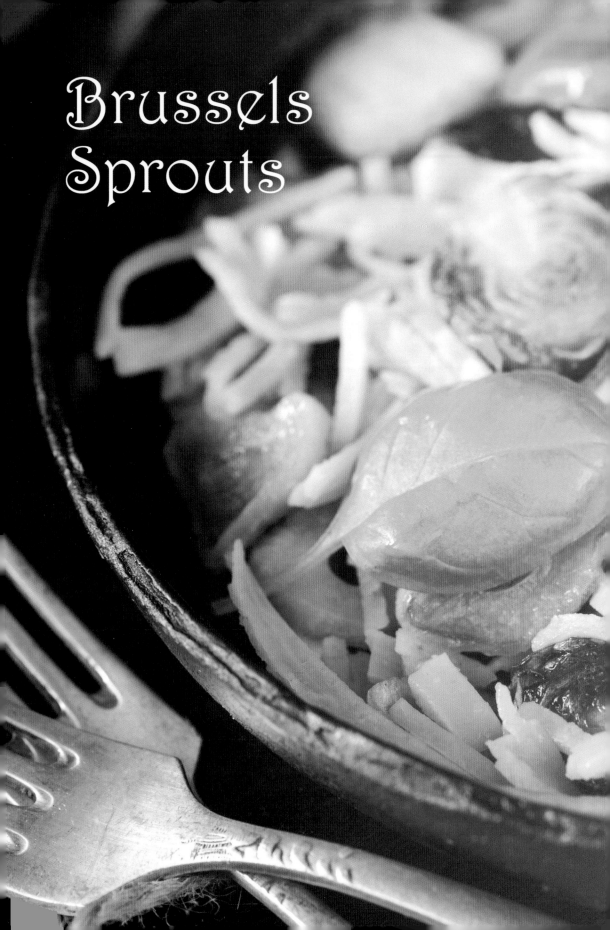

Brussels
Sprouts

Pasta with Roasted Cauliflower and Brussels Sprouts

Ingredients

¾lb of penne or another form of short pasta

½ a cauliflower head cut into florets

8oz Brussels sprouts trimmed and halved

1 medium red onion cut into wedges

4 tablespoons olive oil

2 sprigs of fresh thyme

2oz grated parmesan

Salt and pepper

Heat the oven to 210°C.

Cook the pasta according to its instructions, drain reserving one cup of the water then return to the pan.

In a bowl, toss the sprouts, cauliflower, thyme, onion, salt and pepper and two tablespoons of olive oil then spread out onto two baking sheets.

Roast in the oven until tender and golden brown – for around 25 minutes.

Tip the vegetables into the pan with the pasta, add the remaining tablespoons of oil, a little of the reserved cooking water until the desired consistency is achieved and add the cheese.

Mix well before serving into bowls. Sprinkle with extra cheese if required.

Admittedly Brussels sprouts do not have a reputation as being one of the most loved vegetables on the planet and I have a clear memory of the agony of being forced to eat them as a child, yet now I love them. In Chinese medicine, they are prescribed to help with digestion and they provide support to the body's detox, anti-inflammatory and antioxidant systems. Rich in vitamins A, K, C, B6, folate, potassium, fibre, iron, magnesium and calcium, it is claimed that Brussels sprouts increase male virility. The fibre related nutrients they contain bind with intestinal bile, removing it from the body more effectively thus causing the body to tap into cholesterol supplies to create more bile which results in the lowering of overall cholesterol. A recent study showed that steamed Brussels sprouts bound 27 times more bile than a well-known prescribed cholesterol lowering drug.

Uses – Don't wait until Christmas Day to bring out your Brussels sprouts, instead try them sautéed with balsamic and toasted almonds, shred them and stir fry, cook them with eggs or simply steam them until cooked to perfection, and vibrant green.

Interesting Fact – When combined with wholegrains, sprouts make a complete protein making them a fantastic addition to vegetarian diets.

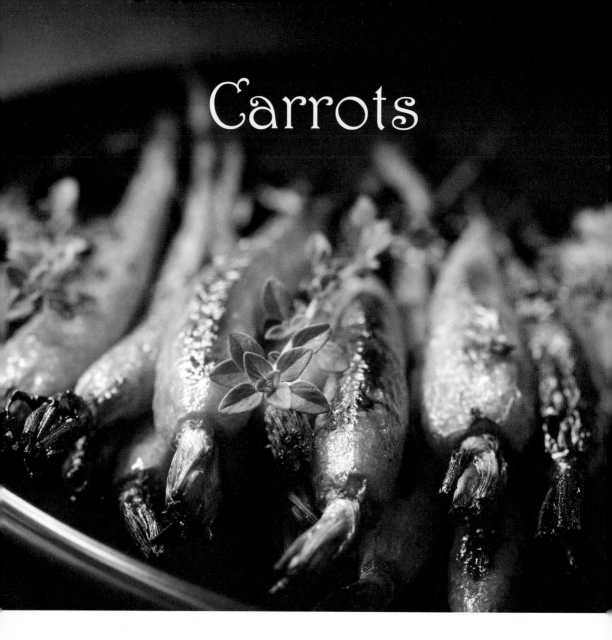

Carrots

Our grandparents may have told us to eat our carrots so that we will be able to see in the dark – what a crazy old wives' tale, or is it? Well it turns out that our grandparents were probably right as carrots are super rich in beta carotene (given away by their bright orange colour) which is turned into vitamin A in the liver. This in turn is transformed in the retina into rhodopsin – a pigment necessary for night vision. Beta carotene has also been shown to prevent the degeneration of the eyes and the development of cataracts. In fact, a study showed that people who consumed large quantities of beta carotene had a 40 per cent lower risk of eye trouble. The high beta carotene content also reduces cell damage and therefore helps to slow down ageing and promote healthier skin – in fact freshly grated carrot is a great homemade face mask. Effective in flushing toxins from the body, the fibre content in carrots helps to promote a healthy colon and digestive system. And that's not all. Regular carrot consumption has been shown to reduce cholesterol levels and therefore may promote heart health. Their potassium content also helps to relax

Carrot, Raisin and Coconut Salad

Ingredients

3 large carrots shredded
1 cup raisins
1 cup walnuts
¼ a cup of finely chopped celery
2 tablespoons shredded coconut

½ cup of mayonnaise
2 tablespoons sour cream
1 tablespoon of cider vinegar
Salt and pepper to season

In a bowl, combine the carrot, raisins, walnuts, coconut and celery.

In a separate jug, whisk together the mayonnaise, sour cream, vinegar and a little salt and pepper.

Add the dressing to the carrot mixture and stir well. Place in the fridge for a couple or hours prior to serving.

the blood vessels and arteries, increasing blood flow and oxygen, and aiding a healthy blood pressure. An excellent source of vitamin C with their antibacterial and antiseptic properties, carrots provide an excellent support to the immune system. Carrots are also hailed for their ability to regulate blood sugar as the carotenoids they contain affect insulin resistance and as a result, lower blood sugar- a must for any diabetic. Carrots are even good for our teeth – yes really! Carrots act like a toothbrush scraping away plaque and food particles and stimulating saliva, this then prevents bacteria which can lead to cavities. And what a fact to end on – a Harvard University study showed that people who ate five or more carrots each week were less likely to suffer a stroke than those who only ate one carrot once a month or less.

Uses – I could write a whole book just dedicated to the use of carrots. I put them in my fresh juice every single day. They are delicious glazed with either honey or balsamic, they make a fantastic mash with parsnips, and are great added to casseroles and stews. Carrot soup is always popular as is homemade coleslaw. I never make a salad without adding grated carrot and carrots are an easy way to hide vegetables in pasta sauces!

Interesting Fact – Whilst we all know carrots as the bright orange, sweet and crunchy vegetable; purple, white, yellow and red carrots do exist too. Plus there are over 100 species of carrots. The word carrot actually comes from the Greek word Karoton – the beta carotene found in carrots was named exactly for that reason.

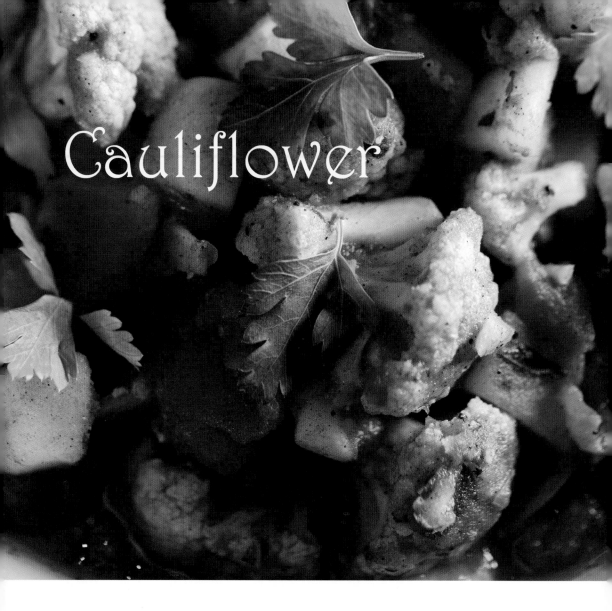

Cauliflower

While cauliflower is thought to have originated from the Mediterranean region some two thousand years ago, a large scale study called the European Prospective Investigation into Cancer and Nutrition (EPIC) has shown that it is now the most commonly eaten cruciferous vegetable in 10 Western European countries. Cauliflower is a popular vegetable, both cooked and raw, although cooked cauliflower binds better with bile acids (which helps to lower cholesterol). Rich in phytonutrients (which help to reduce inflammation) and antioxidants, and bursting with vitamin C as well as being a good source of B vitamins and vitamin K and fibre too, one cup of cauliflower contains around 27 calories When cooked, cauliflower gives off a rather pungent smell which are the natural compounds, or glusosinolates, it contains being released. These glucosinolates are what kick start the body's detoxification system and they have also been shown to prevent certain types of cancer.

Uses – Whilst white cauliflower is the most common, it is also available in purple, green and orange. Due to the recent boom in low carb diets, cauliflower has become a rather fashionable vegetable and is now available in supermarkets in the form of 'cauliflower

Cauliflower Lentil Curry

Ingredients

2 teaspoons of extra virgin olive oil
1 small onion finely chopped
2 garlic cloves minced
I fresh green chilli seeded and
    chopped finely
¾ teaspoon of ground cumin
¾ teaspoon of ground coriander
¼ teaspoon ground turmeric
1 teaspoon of coarse salt

1 tablespoon of tomato pasta
1 cup of dried red lentils
1 medium russet potato peeled and
    chopped into ½ inch pieces
1¾ cups of chicken or vegetable
    stock
½ cup of water
2 cups of cooked jasmine rice
Lime wedges for garnish

Heat the oil in a saucepan on a high heat and cook the onion, garlic and chilli until the onion is soft so for approximately four to five minutes.

Add all the spices and salt and cook for a further two minutes, stirring continuously.

Stir in the tomato paste, lentils, potato, cauliflower, water and stock and bring to a boil.

Reduce the heat, cover and simmer for around 20 minutes until the lentils are soft, check during this cooking time as you may need to add a little more water.

Remove from the heat and leave covered for a further 10 minutes. Serve with the jasmine rice, garnish with lime wedges and maybe a little sliced cucumber.

rice' which is basically grated or finely chopped cauliflower. It really does have so many uses but a few of our favourites include cauliflower soup, cauliflower gratin and we really love it simply roasted. Try to avoid boiling the cauliflower though, as studies have shown that it loses a much greater percentage of nutrients when boiled as opposed to using other cooking methods such as steaming, roasting or sautéing.

Interesting tip – To keep cauliflower looking crisp white add a little lemon ju´ or even milk to it whilst cooking. Cauliflower can be frozen and will retai nutrient content for up to one year.

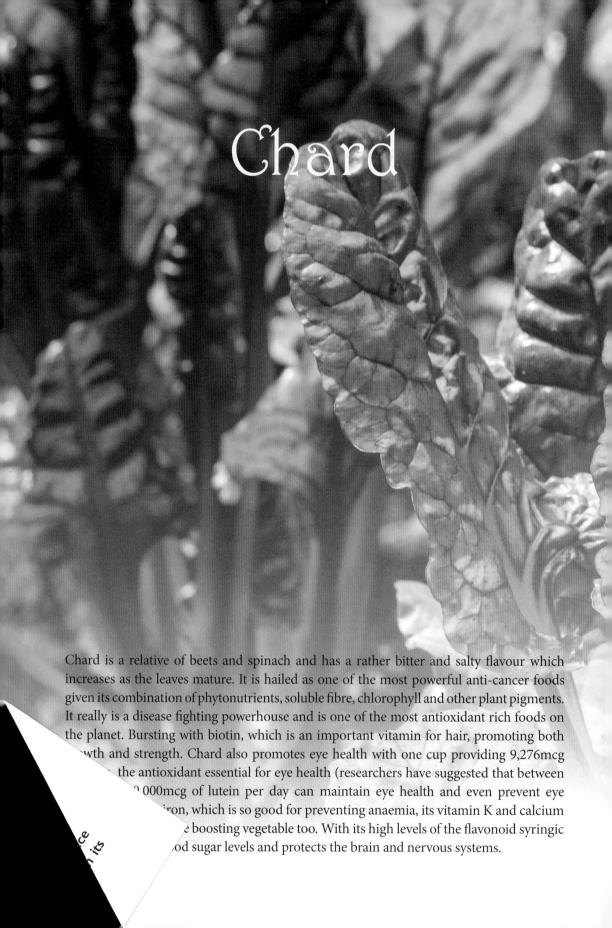

Chard

Chard is a relative of beets and spinach and has a rather bitter and salty flavour which increases as the leaves mature. It is hailed as one of the most powerful anti-cancer foods given its combination of phytonutrients, soluble fibre, chlorophyll and other plant pigments. It really is a disease fighting powerhouse and is one of the most antioxidant rich foods on the planet. Bursting with biotin, which is an important vitamin for hair, promoting both growth and strength. Chard also promotes eye health with one cup providing 9,276mcg ...... the antioxidant essential for eye health (researchers have suggested that between ......000mcg of lutein per day can maintain eye health and even prevent eye ......iron, which is so good for preventing anaemia, its vitamin K and calcium ...... boosting vegetable too. With its high levels of the flavonoid syringic ......od sugar levels and protects the brain and nervous systems.

Swiss Chard with Toasted Breadcrumbs

Ingredients

2½ tablespoons of butter
½ a cup of fresh breadcrumbs

2lb of chard sliced diagonally ¾ inch thickness stems and greens separated
Salt and pepper

Melt half a tablespoon of butter over a medium heat in a large pan and add the fresh breadcrumbs with a pinch of salt and pepper.

Cook whilst stirring for two to three minutes until golden brown then place in a bowl.

Wipe the pan and add the two remaining tablespoons of butter and melt over a medium to high heat.

Cook the stems for four to six minutes until tender, stirring continuously before adding the greens to the pan.

Cover the pan and leave on a low heat for approximately five minutes until the greens are wilted.

Uncover and increase the heat and cook whilst stirring until the pan is dry for approximately eight further minutes. Place into a serving dish, season with salt and pepper and top with the breadcrumbs.

Uses – Although the leaves can be eaten raw in salads the tougher stalks have to be coked separately as they take longer to soften. Briefly boiling or sautéing maintains the most nutrients.

Interesting Fact – Although it is called Swiss Chard it actually originates from Sicily and remains an important ingredient in many Italian and Mediterranean dishes.

Garlic

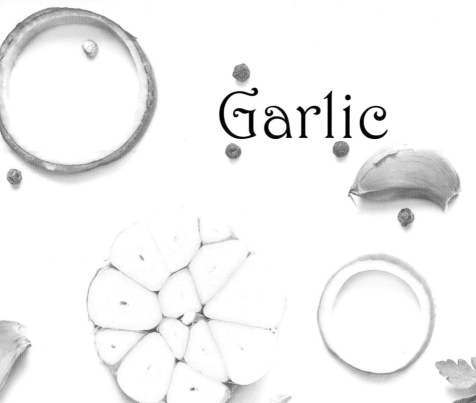

Yes, garlic is classed as a vegetable although many people presume it to be a herb or a spice given that it isn't eaten on its own. Garlic has long been recognized for its medicinal uses. As far back as the ancient times, it was believed that its pungent smell provided strength and courage to those who ate it and it was used for warding off evil spirits and also for embalming. While I can neither deny nor confirm its ability to do any of the above, our ancestors did realize garlic had other healing powers and health benefits and used it to treat everything from colds and infections to broken bones. Garlic is extremely popular across the world and is most famous for its strong flavour and smell owing to its sulphur compounds. Garlic belongs to the same family as onions and leeks – the Lily family. Like onions and leeks, when garlic is sliced or chopped, it releases its sulphur-based enzyme and its smell. The more you slice, grate or mince your garlic the more of the enzyme and antioxidant known as allicin is released.

Garlic has been shown to boost the immune system, and a recent study revealed that people who consumed garlic daily had 63 per cent fewer colds than those who didn't, and not only that, the length of their cold symptoms was also substantially reduced from five days to just one and a half days. Its oxidant content may prevent dementia and Alzheimer's disease, and it has been proven to lower both cholesterol and blood pressure too. In fact, one study from King Khalid University in Saudi Arabia showed that aged garlic extract at doses of 600-1500mg over a 24 week period were just as effective as the drug Atenol at reducing blood pressure. Garlic was one of the very first performance enhancing substances and it is thought that it reduces exercise induced fatigue. There are excellent indications that garlic may promote bone health in women by increasing oestrogen levels and it has also shown positive effects in treating arthritis. Garlic is low in calories but also super rich in vitamin C, B6 and manganese.

Lemon Garlic Fish

Ingredients

4 skinless white fish fillets (6-8oz) about 1 inch in thickness

4 tablespoons of butter (room temperature)

Juice and zest of ½ a lemon

½ teaspoon of dried mixed herbs

3 cloves of garlic minced

4 tablespoons of dry white wine

Salt and pepper

Lemon for garnish

Pinch of red pepper flake

1lb of asparagus with the ends trimmed

Cut four pieces of foil around 12 inches square. Divide the asparagus between the foil, season with salt and pepper then top with a lemon slice.

In a bowl, combine the butter, lemon zest and juice, pepper flakes, salt and pepper, herbs and garlic before placing one tablespoon of the mixture on top of each fish fillet. Place one fish filet onto each foil on top of the asparagus and one tablespoon of wine over each piece – season a little more if required.

Wrap each fish well in the foil and place in the oven for approximately 15 to 20 minutes. Once cooked, carefully remove the fish and place on a plate before pouring over the juices. Serve with lemon slices.

Uses – Garlic definitely isn't confined to garlic bread. But here are a few ideas you may not have thought of. Toss broccoli florets with salt and pepper, olive oil and garlic and roast for the perfect side dish to any meal, sauté peas with garlic and onion, or make the most delicious dip to impress your guests with blue cheese, garlic and bacon.

Take note – Whilst some vegetables contain many nutrients in their skins, the skin of garlic is inedible. Also, the pungent smell and taste of garlic is reduced the longer it is cooked so if you prefer a milder dish, cook it a little longer. But beware, if you overcook it, it will taste bitter.

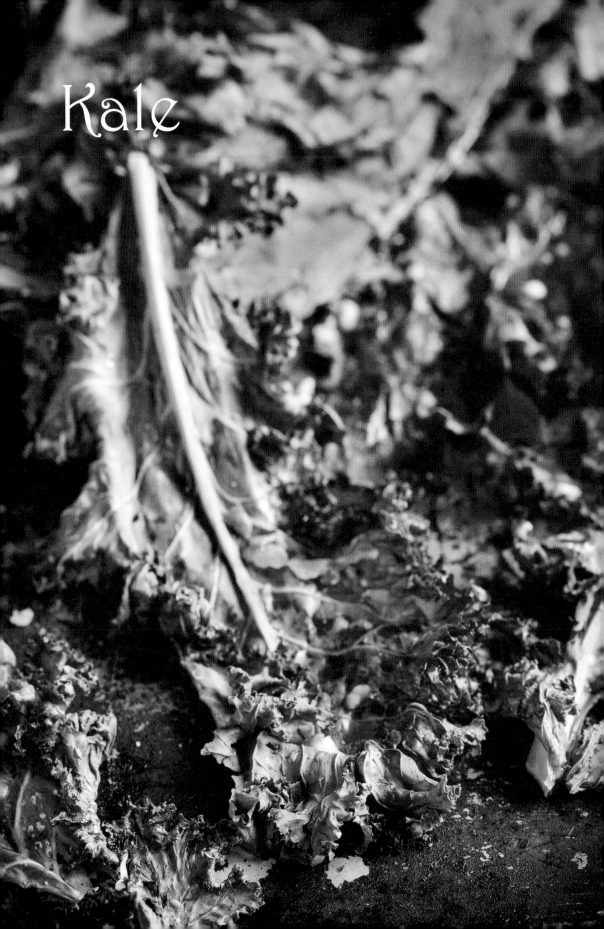

Kale

Kale Chips

Ingredients

A bunch of kale   1 teaspoon of salt
1 tablespoon olive oil

Preheat the oven to 175°C and line a baking tray with greaseproof paper.

Remove the kale leaves from the thick stems and tear into bite size pieces, then wash and dry well.

Lay on the baking tray, drizzle with the olive oil and sprinkle with salt.

Bake for between 10 and 15 minutes until the edges are brown but not burnt and the kale is crispy. You can add other seasoning if you wish.

Not all that long ago, most people would not have even have heard of kale and then it exploded onto the superfood scene and gained a host of followers and devotees praising its potent nutrient content and health benefits. I have to admit I am one of those devotees! A member of the cabbage family and one of the most nutrient dense vegetables or even foods on the planet, it has powerful, medicinal properties. A single cup of raw kale has only 33 calories yet it contains 206 per cent of the recommended daily allowance (RDA) of vitamin A, 684 per cent RDA of vitamin K, 134 per cent RDA of vitamin C, nine per cent RDA of vitamin B6, 26 per cent RDA of manganese, nine per cent RDA of calcium, 10 per cent RDA of copper, nine per cent RDA of potassium and six per cent of magnesium.

Like most leafy greens, it is high in antioxidants which counter the damage to the by from free radicals. Kale also has anti-inflammatory, anti-bacterial, anti-depressant properties and is much richer in vitamin C than most vegetables, boasting five times the amount found in spinach, and even more than an orange per cup. Kale is one of the best possible sources of vitamin K, contains numerous cancer fighting substances such as sulforphane and is a great source of beta carotene.

Uses – Kale works fabulously in stews, soups and casseroles, and I add it to my smoothies but best of all, are homemade kale chips seasoned simply with olive oil and sea salt. What are you waiting for?

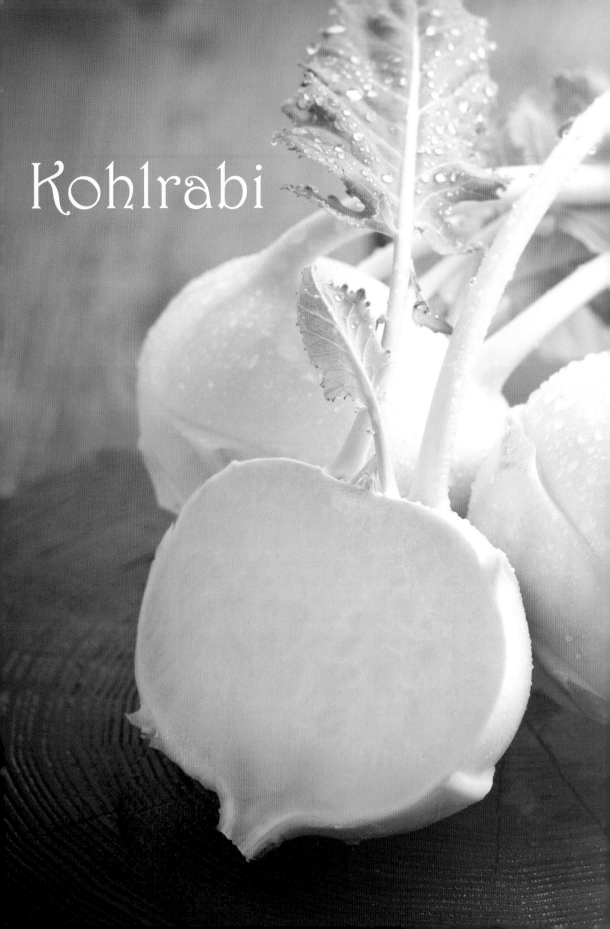

Kohlrabi

Kohlrabi Chips

Ingredients

Very thinly sliced kohlrabi   Sea salt
Olive oil

Preheat the oven to 250°C degrees and line a baking tray with greaseproof paper.

Toss the kohlrabi in the olive oil and season with salt. Place in a single layer on the baking sheet and bake in the oven for around 45 minutes until crisp and golden.

Transfer to a plate and season with a little more salt.

This alien looking vegetable comes from the same family as cabbage, broccoli and cauliflower and its name in German translates to 'turnip'. It is particularly popular in India. The whole of the vegetable is edible although the bulbous bottom is the most common part to eat. Surprisingly delicious raw, both sweet and peppery, kohlrabi is super rich in phytonutrients, which you now know are essential for cancer prevention and are also a great liver detoxifier. Bursting with vitamin C, with just one cup proving us with 140 per cent of our recommended intake, kohrabi can therefore boost the immune system and aid the absorption of iron. A fantastic source of fibre and potassium, this vegetable helps to promote healthy intestines and also aids the regulation of blood pressure.

Uses – Given that it tastes so good raw, kohlrabi is a good addition to salads, and works well as a crudité with dips but it is delicious cubed and roasted then served as a lovely sweet and caramelized addition to meat of fish too. It can also be steamed or stir fried.

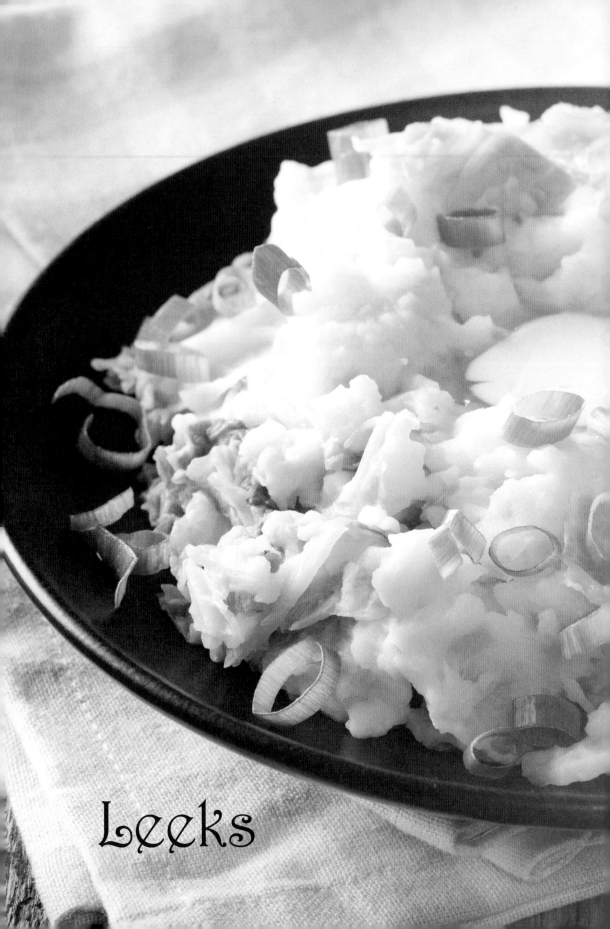

Leeks

Colcannon

This recipe is originally from County Mayo and having an Irish mother often made it onto our dining table and was always popular.

Ingredients

1lb pound cabbage	1 cup of milk
1lb potato	½ cup of butter
2 leeks chopped	Salt and pepper

In separate pans, boil the cabbage and potatoes until tender, and then drain and chop them both, keeping the potatoes warm.

In a third pan, simmer the leeks in the milk until tender. Season the potatoes then mash. Add in the leeks and the milk before adding in the chopped cabbage. Pour in the melted butter and mix well.

Leeks have a distinct flavour but it is much more delicate than those of its family members of onions and shallots. When sliced or chopped, the antioxidants in leeks begin to convert into allicin. Allicin is highly antibacterial, antiviral and antifungal. It lowers cholesterol by impeding harmful enzymes in liver cells. One serving provides more than half of our daily requirement of vitamin K and more than a quarter of our requirement of vitamin A. Leeks contain high amounts of niacin, riboflavin, folic acid, magnesium and thiamine, making them an excellent bone food and also a wise choice for pregnant women. Leeks have been proven to have diuretic, laxative and antiseptic properties; they contain cancer fighting compounds and support the heart and blood supply system. They are also low in calories and a good source of soluble and insoluble fibre.

Uses – I am sure everyone will have enjoyed a leek based soup at some point and colcannon is also an old favourite, but try adding leeks to quiches, stir fries, roasting them or add to potatoes for a twist on a gratin.

Interesting Fact – Leek has been the national symbol of Wales for more than 700 years and they are one of the world's oldest known vegetables.

Onion

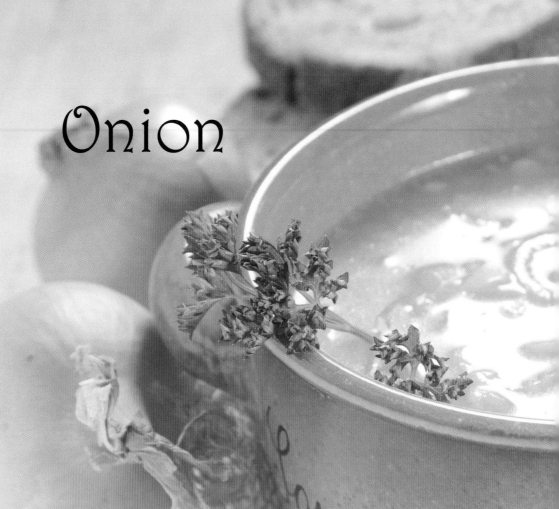

So I thought I would stick with the Lily family and move straight onto the onion which has many similar health benefits to garlic with its allicin content. The compounds in onions become airborne when sliced or diced which is the reason chopping onions is usually a tearful experience – and painful – it can really sting! But believe me, it is worth it. There are three types of onions, red, white and yellow and they are excellent sources of vitamin C, sulphuric compounds, phytonutrients and flavonoids. Many studies over the years have shown that flavonoids may help to reduce the risk of many illnesses and diseases such as Parkinson's disease, stroke and heart disease. Quercetin is a flavonoid contained in onions that has been linked to preventing cancer by acting as an antioxidant. It is also praised for preventing bladder infections and lowering blood pressure as well as relaxing the muscles in the airways thus reducing asthma symptoms.

It is the high levels of antioxidants in onions that give them their lovely sweet flavour and aroma and these very antioxidants are thought to reduce inflammation and promote a healthy heart. Onions contain fibre, promoting a healthy digestive system and colon. A good source of chromium means that onions help to regulate blood sugar and are therefore particularly helpful to diabetes sufferers. Onions may even improve the bone density of post- menopausal women as a 2009 study in the journal *Menopause* found that daily consumption improved bone density and reduced the risk of hip fracture by 20 per cent. Onions are low in calories and contain no fat.

Balsamic Glazed Red Onions

Ingredients

4 medium red onions
2 tablespoons olive oil
2 tablespoons balsamic

1½ tablespoons of chopped oregano
Large pinch of salt and cracked black pepper

To Glaze:
1 tablespoon of balsamic vinegar
1 teaspoon of Dijon mustard

2 tablespoons of olive oil
Large pinch of salt and pepper

Preheat the oven to 200°C

Slice the onions in half and remove the paper skins then cut each half into four wedges keeping the root centre intact.

Pack the wedges tightly into an ovenproof dish (a 9 inch round oval dish works well with this).

Sprinkle over the olive oil, balsamic, one tablespoon of the oregano and salt and pepper – no need to stir.

Cover with foil and place in the oven for 30 minutes. Remove the foil and cook for a further 30 minutes uncovered.

In a separate bowl, whisk the balsamic, mustard, salt and pepper then gradually add the olive oil. Pour the glaze over the roasted onions and place back in the oven for a further 10 minutes.

Remove from the oven, sprinkle with the remaining oregano and serve.

Uses – A truly super, versatile vegetable that can be eaten either cooked or raw, onions can be used in salads, stews and casseroles. They are also great in dips or tarts and roasted with balsamic. My all-time favourite is traditional French onion soup, which I first remember tasting in a restaurant on holiday as a child. It really doesn't get any better!

Top tip – There is a huge concentration of flavonoids in the outer layers of the onion so try to maintain as much of these when peeling.

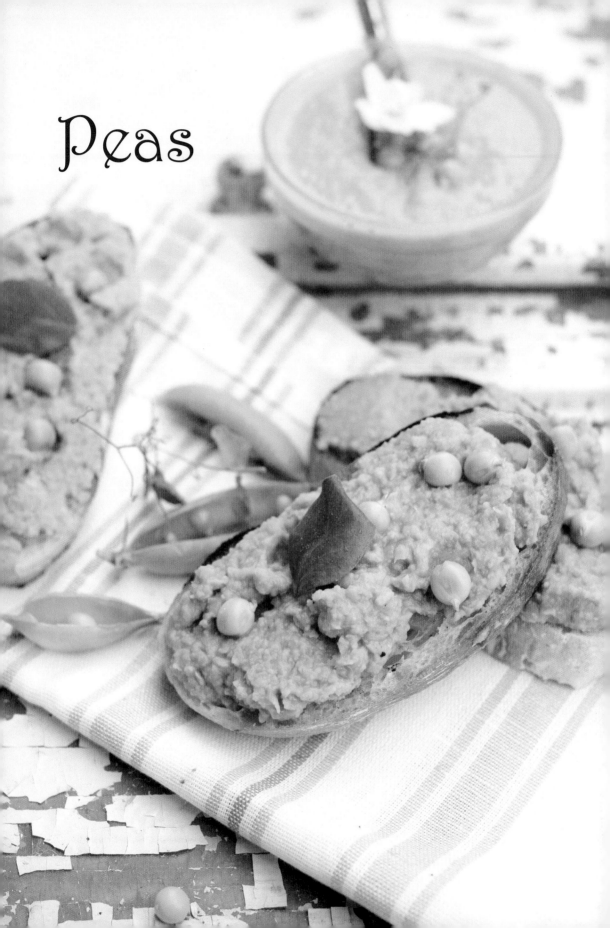

Peas

Pea, Pancetta and Potato salad

Ingredients

800g baby new potatoes
300g frozen green peas
Juice of half a lemon

140g pancetta cubes
Handful basil
Handful mint

Cook the potatoes in a large pan of boiling water until tender – around 12 to 15 minutes.

Add the peas for the last couple of minutes of cooking, then drain. During this time, fry the pancetta until crisp, remove from the heat then add the lemon juice and salt and pepper.

Add the potatoes, peas, basil and mint to the pan, stir well and serve. This is delicious both hot and cold.

I adore peas! These little balls of goodness are bursting with vitamins and minerals. They are excellent source of vitamins C, K, B1 and folate, are virtually fat free and have a surprisingly high protein content with 100g providing 5.42g. A super bone healthy vegetable, the B vitamins help to metabolize both carbohydrates and proteins, making peas the perfect energy boosting vegetable too.

Uses – Peas not only make a great side dish but they can easily take centre stage in many recipes. They work well with rice – pea and spring vegetable risotto is divine. I make a delicious pea soup which my whole family loves and mushy peas never fail to bring a smile to my children's faces.

Interesting Fact – The Chinese were the first to taste this vegetable around 2000 BC, peas are mentioned in the bible and we are led to believe they were worshipped in Rome, Egypt and Greece.

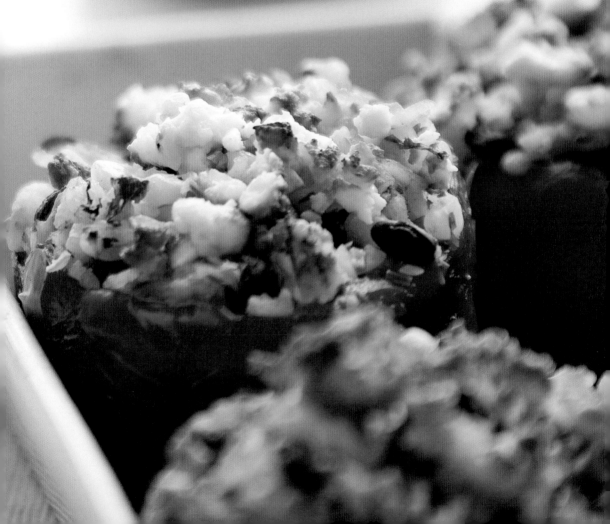

Red Pepper

Baked Stuffed Red Peppers

Ingredients

2 red bell peppers halved
  lengthways
   with the core, stem and seeds
   removed
1 cup cherry tomatoes
1½oz feta cheese crumbled

1 teaspoon of thyme chopped
8 basil leaves torn into pieces
1 tablespoon of extra virgin olive
  oil
Pepper to season

Preheat the oven to 200°C. Place the bell peppers in an oven proof dish with the core side facing upwards.

In a bowl, toss together the feta, thyme, tomatoes and basil and load into the peppers. Drizzle with olive oil then bake in the oven covered with foil for around 30 minutes until the peppers begin to soften.

Remove the foil and bake for a further 10 to 15 minutes until the skins of the tomatoes begin to burst and the cheese starts to turn golden and toasted.

Serve with a fresh green salad.

Because green peppers are not fully mature, they have a much lower vitamin content than the red variety. The most nutritious red peppers are those with the brightest skin which is shiny and tight to the touch. Red peppers contain more than 200 per cent of your daily vitamin C requirement and are an excellent source of vitamin B6 and folate, both of which can help to prevent anaemia. Packed with antioxidants, they have one of the highest concentrations of lycopene of any vegetable. Their vitamin A content helps to support healthy vision and they have a thermogenic action which means they can increase metabolism, resulting in more calories being burned. The list of their uses is endless but popular recipes in our house are red pepper omelette, stuffed peppers and roasted peppers.

Interesting Fact – Red peppers are actually green bell peppers that have been harvested and matured until they take on a deep red colour and have a milder and sweeter flavour.

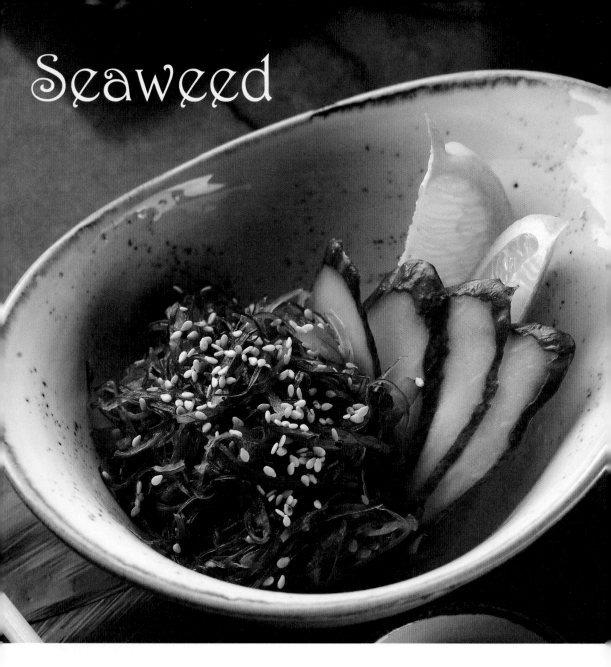

Seaweed

The sea provides us with an amazing array of highly nutritious vegetables. Our ancestors thought seaweed was the key to health and longevity and they ate it daily for optimum nutrition. Seaweed has been considered a perfect food in China for over two thousand years. Some well-known and fairly common seaweeds include kelp, nori, bladder wrack, hijiki, wakame, sea lettuce and dulse. Many are even available in supermarkets now and most definitely in health food stores. Drawing their minerals from the sea, seaweed is rich in iodine, calcium, magnesium, iron, vitamins C and A, B, fibre and protein – containing more vitamins and minerals than most vegetables.

With its strong antiviral, anti-inflammatory and antibacterial properties, the high iodine content in seaweed promotes a healthy thyroid and contains more vitamin C than an orange, boosting the immune system and providing the building blocks for collagen. There is also evidence to suggest that seaweed may also increase our resistance against allergies and infection, aid heart health, digestion, improve liver function and stabilize blood sugar.

Seaweed Risotto

Ingredients

3 tablespoons of olive oil
1 large onion chopped
2 medium shallots chopped
3 cloves garlic chopped
¾ teaspoon sea salt
1 cup of dry white wine – optional
6 cups of vegetable stock
1/3 cup of mascarpone cheese

¼oz of dried nori seaweed toasted
Zest of half a lemon and some juice
½ cup parmesan cheese
1 and a half cups of spinach finely
   chopped
1 cup of toasted walnuts
2 cups of pearled barley

Heat the oil in a large pan over a medium heat and add the onions, shallots, garlic and salt and sauté for around four minutes until the onions are soft.

Add the barley to the pan and cook for a further four minutes until it has a nice sheen.

Add the wine and simmer for three to four minutes until the barley has absorbed a lot of the liquid.

In batches, add the stock, no more than one cupful at a time and wait until that has been absorbed prior to adding the next cup.

This whole process should take approximately 40 minutes – stir regularly to prevent the barley sticking to the bottom of the pan.

Once all of the stock has been added and the barley is tender, remove the pan from the heat and stir in the mascarpone, lemon zest and most of the parmesan.

Next, stir in the seaweed followed by the chopped spinach.

Load into bowls, add a splash of lemon juice, and top with toasted walnuts and a little more parmesan.

Uses – High in protein, low in fat and containing little or no carbohydrates, seaweed works well in salads, is delicious in noodle or miso soup, toast nori strips and use with dips or fill as you would a wrap and seaweed can make a really lovely crust for meat or fish.

Interesting Fact – Seaweed contains fourteen times more calcium by weight than milk.

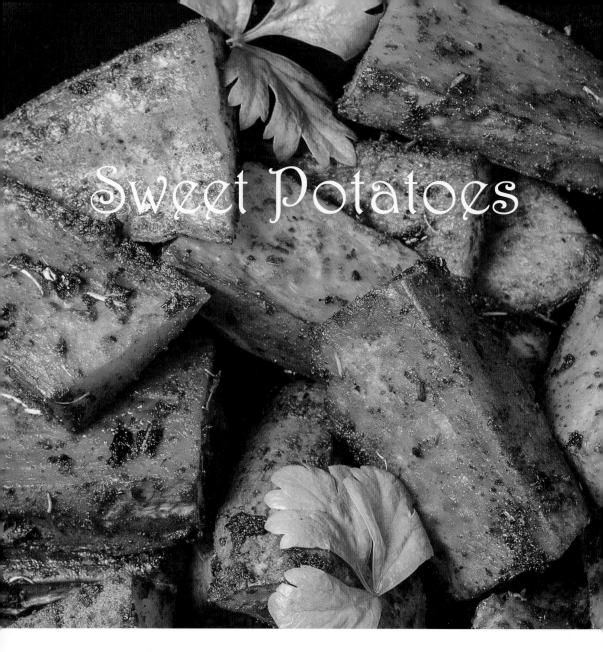

Sweet Potatoes

How sweet is it that sweet potatoes are so good for our health? I often feel that the sweet potato is so undervalued, and yet it is one of the most nutritious foods in the world. Bright orange in colour and rich in both vitamins A and C, vitamin B6, beta carotene and manganese, providing natural anti-inflammatory properties. Once again, the high vitamin C content helps to promote collagen, and the carotenoids in sweet potato may help the body respond to insulin and stabilize blood sugar. Sweet potatoes are also rich in beta cryptoxanthin (a powerful antioxidant) and this has been found to help prevent certain inflammatory diseases such as arthritis. Being a good source of dietary fibre means they promote a healthy digestive system and several studies have shown that the may help to cleanse the body of toxins and heavy metals. They may also help to prevent constipation and sooth the pain of stomach ulcers.

Sweet Potato and Spinach Quesadillas

Ingredients

2 large sweet potatoes
½ a cup of sugar
1 cup of red wine vinegar
1 large red onion sliced
5 cups of baby spinach

1 cup of mozzarella shredded
2 tablespoons of olive oil
8 6-inch tortillas
Salt and pepper
4 black peppercorns

Bake the sweet potatoes in the oven until tender for approximately 45 minutes to one hour.

During this time combine the vinegar, peppercorns and sugar in a saucepan and bring to the boil, stirring until all the sugar has dissolved.

Place the onion in an ovenproof dish and pour the vinegar mixture over and leave to stand for ten minutes.

Drain the onion and transfer to a plate to cool.

Remove the potatoes from the oven and split open with a knife. Remove the soft centre and mash in a bowl seasoning with salt and pepper.

Lay out four tortillas. Divide the sweet potato between them, and add a large handful of spinach, a quarter of a cup of cheese then top with another tortilla.

In a large pan, heat a teaspoon of the oil and in batches, place the tortillas cooking on both sides until they are crisp and the cheese is melted – approximately three minutes on each side.

Cut into quarters and serve with the onions.

Uses – For a start you can simply replace your regular potatoes with sweet potatoes in virtually any dish from shepherd's pie, to roast dinners to a plain jacket potato but for a sin free treat you can make sweet potato fries by scrubbing sweet potatoes (always leave the skins on for maximum nutrient content), slicing into fries, tossing in olive oil, sprinkling with sea salt and roasting in the oven for around 25 to 30 minutes. Be sure to make plenty as these are always super popular!

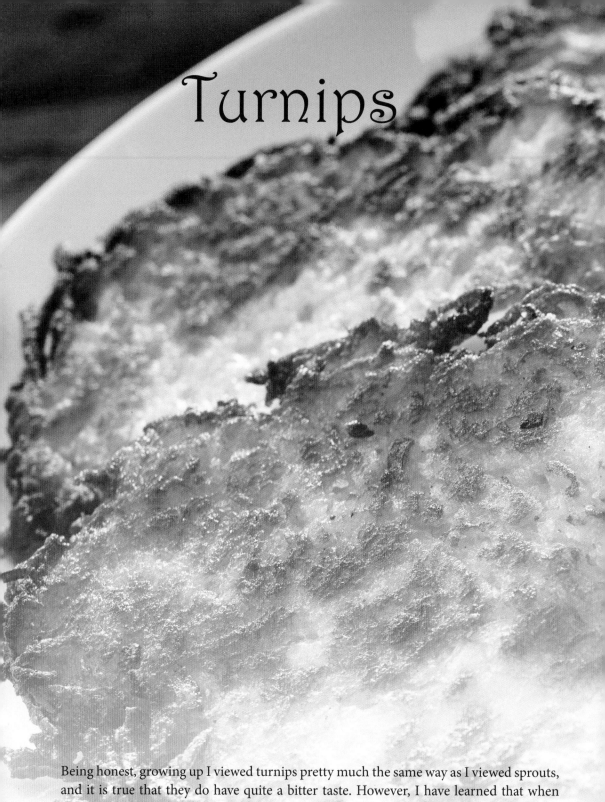

Turnips

Being honest, growing up I viewed turnips pretty much the same way as I viewed sprouts, and it is true that they do have quite a bitter taste. However, I have learned that when cooked and seasoned well turnips can make a dish complete – my root vegetable soup wouldn't be the same without them! Another cruciferous vegetable, turnips have high levels of antioxidants which have been linked to a reduced risk of cancer. Their high

Turnip and Potato Patties

Ingredients

½lb of turnips peeled and cut into
  ¼ inch cubes

6oz of potatoes peeled and cut into
  half an inch cubes

2 to 3 tablespoons of thinly sliced
  scallion greens

1 beaten egg

¼ cup of all-purpose flour

Olive oil

Salt and pepper

In a large pan, boil the turnip and potato until tender, this should take between 15 and 20 minutes. Drain and mash.

Stir in the scallions, egg, flour salt and pepper and mix well.

Add olive oil to a wide bottom pan and heat to a high heat.

Using your hands, take the potato and turnip mixture and mould into patties before placing into the hot pan.

Cook for approximately four minutes on each side until golden.

content of vitamin K and Omega-3 fatty acids makes them natural anti- inflammatories and may also reduce the risk of heart disease. Bursting with vitamins A, C, E plus manganese and beta carotene, they are an excellent source of fibre which promotes a feeling of fullness for longer and so may aid weight loss and also provide for a healthy digestive system. Finally, turnips are a bone healthy food full of calcium, potassium and essential minerals which not only promote healthy bone growth, but which may also prevent bone diseases such as osteoporosis.

Uses – Turnips are so versatile, as you can roast, bake, steam, mash, and boil them. They make a delicious vegetable gratin, are fabulous in soups and a dish of roasted vegetables simply with olive oil and salt and pepper would be bare without them!

Interesting Fact – Both the root of the vegetable and the leaves can be eaten – in fact, the leaves are the most nutritious part.

Watercress

This dark green leaf grows naturally in spring water, hence the name. Watercress is top of the Aggregate Nutrient Density Index which is a measure based on vitamin, mineral and phytonutrient content per calorie. Watercress has the highest possible score of a thousand. More than 70 per cent of studies into the area have found links between cruciferous vegetables such as watercress and the protection against cancer. Cruciferous vegetables contain phytonutrients and according to the National Institute of Cancer these compounds may help to protect cells from DNA damage. They also have antiviral and antibacterial benefits, and inhibit tumour blood vessel formation and tumour cell migration.

Watercress is also an excellent source of those eye-loving nutrients of vitamin A, beta carotene, lutein and zeaxanthin. Lutein and zeaxanthin have shown to be good for people with cardiovascular disease as they can reduce the hardening of the arteries, thus making heart attacks less likely. Watercress also has a high level of nitrates which have a range of heart health benefits. Watercress is good for your bones as just one cup contains your total daily requirement of vitamin K so watercress really does have your bone health all wrapped up in one serving! Bursting with antioxidants and minerals also makes it great for skin health with a recent survey showing that after adding one bag of watercress to their diet daily, 10 out of 11 women reported visible improvements to their skin after just four weeks.

Uses – With its slightly peppery taste, soft leaves and crunchy, edible stalks, watercress is a great addition to salads and smoothies, and watercress soup is not only delicious, it is highly nutritious too.

Interesting Fact – Watercress has more bioavailable calcium (the calcium the body can actually absorb) than milk and even better, watercress does not contain casein which is the often hard to digest protein found in milk so it is easier for the body.

Butternut Squash and Watercress Cannelloni

Ingredients

1 tablespoon olive oil

1 onion chopped

2 cloves garlic minced

675g butternut squash, peeled, seeded and chopped into cubes

1 teaspoon dried sage

150ml dry white wine

200ml vegetable stock

2 85g bags of watercress chopped

25g toasted pine nuts

100g gorgonzola cheese crumbled

1 300g pack of fresh lasagne sheets

1 large 680g jar of passata

50g grated parmesan cheese

1 tablespoon pine nuts

Heat the olive oil in a large frying pan and sauté the onion until golden for around five minutes.

Add the garlic and squash to the pan and cook for only one minute before adding the wine, sage and stock.

Season with salt and pepper then cover and simmer for around 20 minutes until the squash is tender. Drain any excess liquid and reserve.

Mash the squash lightly with a fork then stir in the watercress, gorgonzola, pine nuts and half of the parmesan cheese.

Preheat the oven to 180°C and grease an ovenproof dish.

Lay all the fresh lasagne sheets out flat then divide the mixture between each sheet laying a line of mixture along the edge of one side of each sheet.

Carefully roll the sheets into perfect cannelloni rolls then place with the seam side down into the baking dish. Once all the sheets are in the dish, pour over the passata, sprinkle with the remaining parmesan and pine nuts and bake in the oven for between 25 and30 minutes until it is hot and bubbling and the pasta is tender.

Serve with a watercress salad.

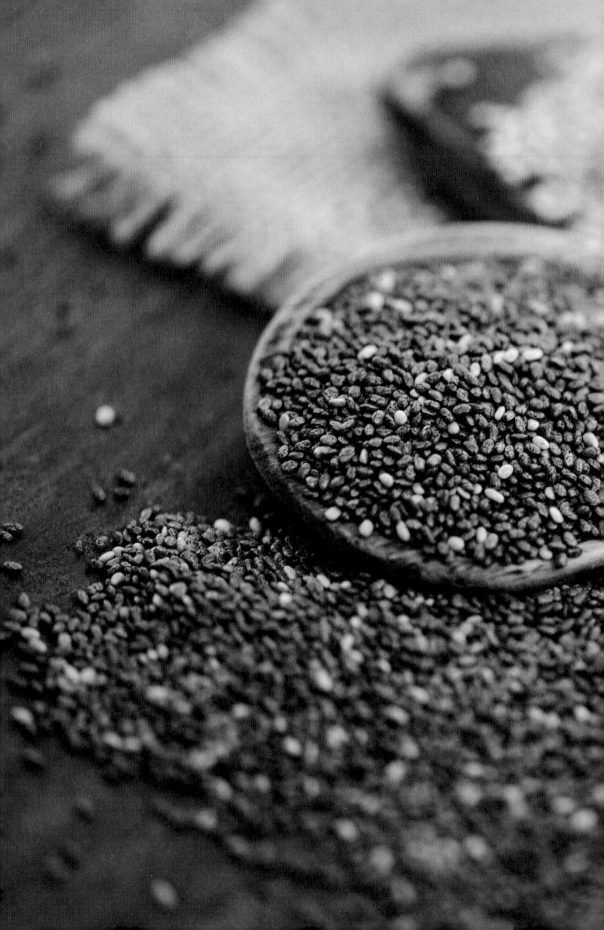

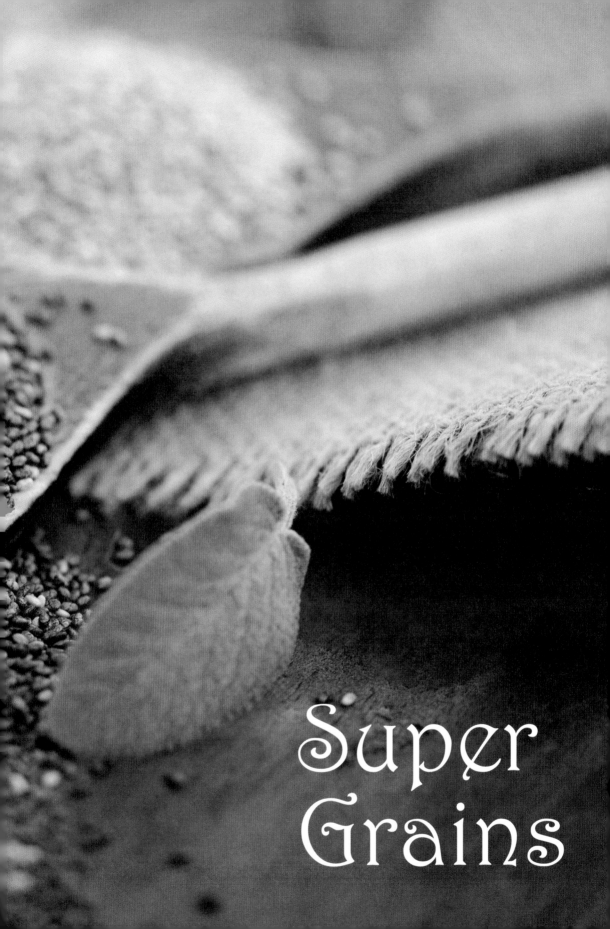

Super
Grains

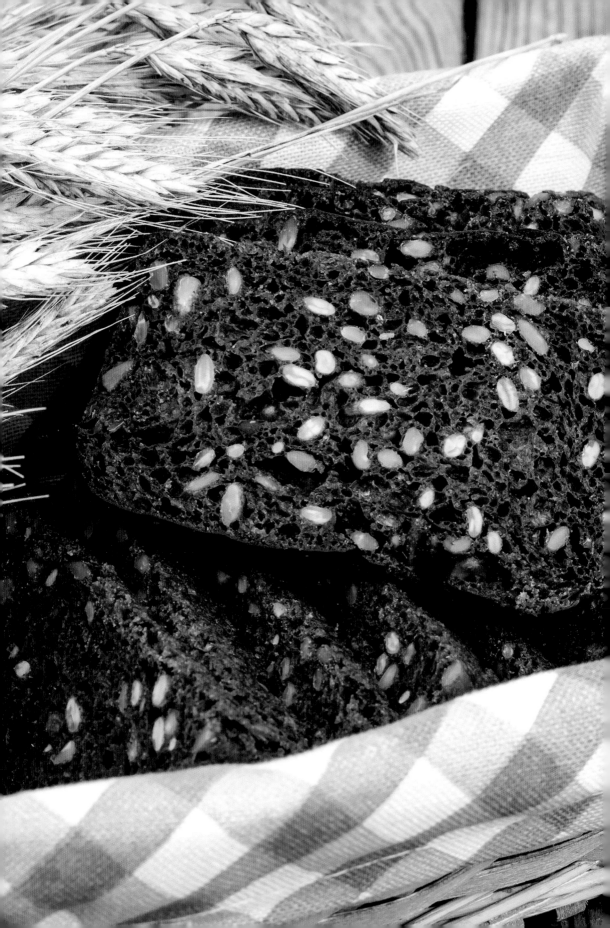

A grain is described in several dictionaries as 'a single, small hard seed, a seed or a fruit of a cereal or grass.' Grains are highly nutritious, delicious and easy to cook, and form a vital part of a healthy diet. Grains can be split into two groups – whole grains and refined grains. Whole grains contain the entire grain kernel so the bran, germ and endosperm (the outer tissue). Examples include whole wheat flour, rolled oats, popcorn, quinoa and brown rice. Refined grains have been milled, which is a process that removes the bran and germ. Whilst this process provides a finer texture and improves shelf life, it also removes fibre, iron and many B vitamins. Examples of refined grains include white rice, couscous and white bread. I have chosen what I consider to be some of the most nutritious grains.

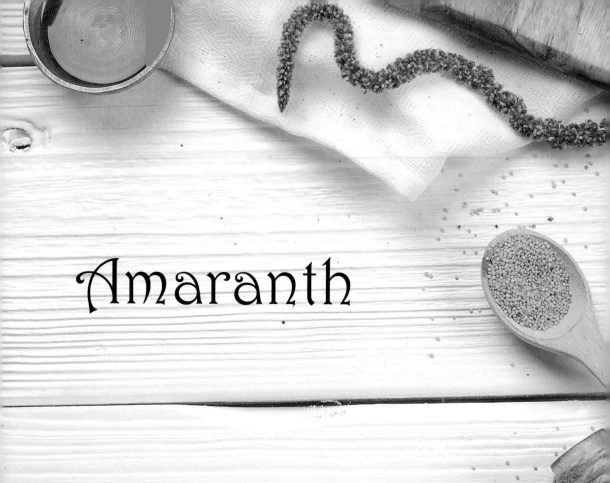

Amaranth

Native to Peru, today amaranth is gown in Africa, China, India and Russia as well as South America. It technically isn't a grain but the fruit of a plant which usually grows to about 6ft and has a sweet, peppery taste. It is rich in vitamins, A, K, B6, C, and also boasts plenty of folate, riboflavin, calcium, potassium, iron, copper, magnesium and manganese. Amaranth is an excellent source of fibre and contains more than 30 per cent protein than wheat flour or oats. It is also another rare source of complete plant protein and is naturally gluten free. It has been shown to reduce cholesterol, blood pressure, inflammation, and to aid the body in absorbing calcium, boosting energy and building muscle. It is also effective in preventing the greying of hair as well as providing an immune boost and aiding the regulation of hormones.

Uses – It can be popped to make popcorn which is always entertaining, and is also a perfect rice or pasta substitute; just cook one cup of amaranth with three cups of water until all the water is absorbed and it is fluffy and light. Try making amaranth rice pudding or use the flour in baking as a gluten free alternative to regular flour.

Interesting Fact – The Aztecs thought that amaranth had super natural powers and used it in their religious ceremonies.

Amaranth with Spinach, Mushroom and Tomato Sauce

Ingredients

1 cup of amaranth
1 tablespoon olive oil
1 bunch or bag of spinach
2 ripe tomatoes skinned and
  chopped

½lb of mushrooms sliced
1½ teaspoons of dried basil
1½ teaspoons of dried oregano
1 clove of garlic minced
½ onion chopped finely
Salt and pepper to season

Add the amaranth to boiling water. Bring back to the boil before reducing the heat and simmering for approximately 20 minutes.

Meanwhile heat the oil in the pan and add the garlic and onion and cook for approximately four minutes until softened.

Add the tomatoes, onions, basil, oregano, spinach, salt and pepper and a tablespoon of water and cook for around 15 minutes, crushing the tomatoes when stirring.

Drain the amaranth. This can be served with the sauce stirred into the amaranth or simply poured on top.

Barley

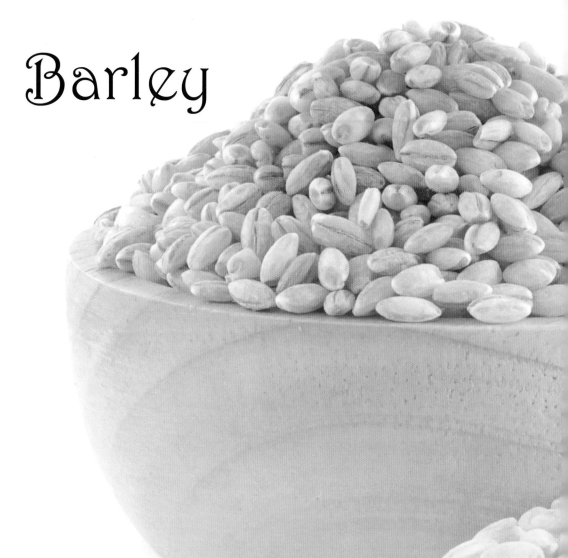

Barley is one of the oldest consumed grains in the world, and while it may not be as popular as oats, wheat or even quinoa, it contains the lowest amount of fat and calories and the highest amount of fibre of all the grains. It originated in Western Asia and Northeast Africa and was the staple grain of peasants during medieval times. Just one cup of barley contains around 6g of fibre and it is the insoluble type which is associated with promoting heart health, reducing cholesterol, balancing blood sugar levels, aiding weight loss by promoting a feeling of fullness and preventing cravings, aiding a healthy digestive system and preventing constipation. Rich in antioxidants and bursting with the minerals magnesium, calcium, folate, potassium, copper, niacin, thiamine, selenium and manganese, which help to promote healthy skin, hair and nails, it also supports the nervous system by aiding muscle function, regulating hormones and helping to prevent certain cancers. Consuming barley has been shown to prevent the formation of gallstones whilst its phosphorous and copper content ensure good bone formation and prevent the risk of fractures.

Grilled and Stuffed Barley Portabellas

Ingredients

½ a cup of uncooked pearl barley

1 tablespoon of olive oil

10 small white mushrooms finely chopped

5 basil leaves finely chopped

2 cloves of garlic minced

1 courgette finely chopped

1 red onion finely chopped

1 red bell pepper finely chopped

8 large portabella mushrooms

1 tablespoon Dijon mustard mixed with 2 tablespoons of olive oil

Salt and pepper to season

½ a cup of toasted pecans

Bring one and a half cups of water to the boil, add the barley then return to the boil. Reduce the heat, cover and simmer for 35 minutes.

Meanwhile, in a large pan heat the oil over a medium to high heat and add the mushrooms, basil, courgette, onion, garlic, bell pepper and a little salt and pepper and cook for 10 to 15 minutes, stirring occasionally.

Once the barley has cooked, drain and add to the vegetables. Brush the portabellas with the mustard and olive oil and place under a grill stalk side down for 8 to10 minutes.

Turn and fill each portabella with the vegetable mixture before placing them back under the grill for a further five minutes. Serve with a green salad and a little extra vegetable mix on the side.

Uses – Barley is commonly used to make animal feed as well as drinks such as beer and wine, barley water and barley tea. My mother always added barley to her homemade soups when I was a child but it has many other uses. Try making barley risotto, using it to make homemade burgers or adding barley to stews and salads. **Barley does contain gluten and therefore is not a suitable choice for those with coeliac disease or for people who are gluten intolerant.**

Interesting Fact – In a 2007 ranking of grains grown around the world, barley came in fourth place with 136 million tonnes grown every year.

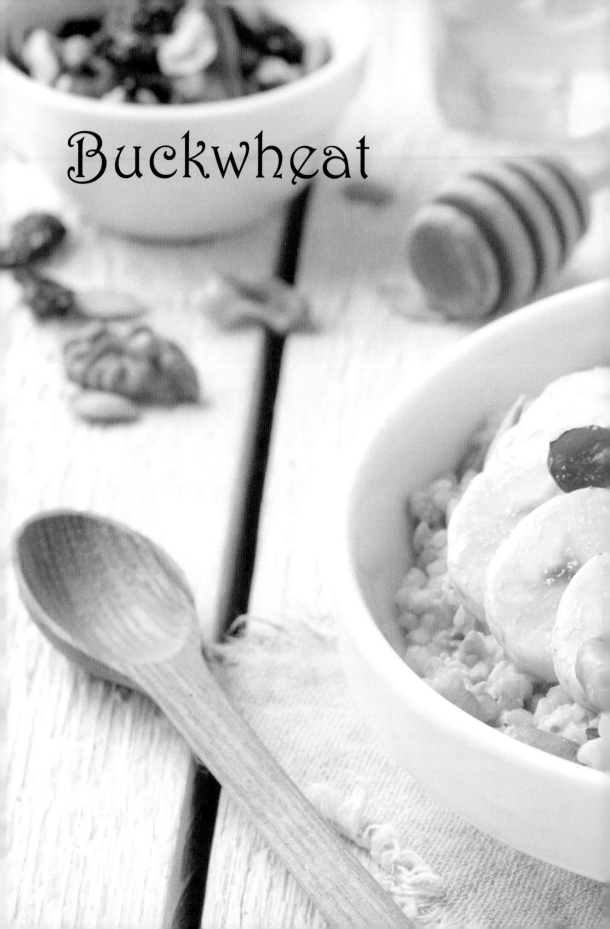

Buckwheat

Buckwheat Granola

Ingredients

2 cups of rolled oats
¾ cup of buckwheat groats chopped
¾ cup sunflower seeds
Pinch of salt
3 tablespoons of coconut oil

¼ of a cup of honey
½ a cup of almonds chopped
1 vanilla bean split and chopped
½ a cup of flaked coconut
½ a cup of raisins

Preheat the oven to 150°C and line a baking tray with greaseproof paper.

Mix the oats, buckwheat sunflower seeds and salt in a large bowl.

Place a small saucepan over a medium heat and melt the coconut oil.

Add the honey and the vanilla pod seeds and mix until you have a smooth runny liquid. Pour this liquid over the oat mixture and mix well before spreading onto the baking tray.

Bake in the oven for 35 to 40 minutes, stirring the mixture every 10 minutes.

Stir in the almonds and bake for five to ten minutes more.

Remove from the oven and allow to cool completely before adding in the raisins and coconut.

This is not just a delicious breakfast but a perfect any time of day snack.

The seed of a flowering herb plant that grows to around 60cm in height, it has more starch and less fat than other seeds and is known for its lovely, buttery taste. First cultivated in South Eastern China and the Himalayas where it was a staple food for many years, buckwheat is an excellent source of energy, and although it contains substantially less protein than quinoa, it contains an excellent range of amino acids. Naturally gluten free, it can help to lower cholesterol and to remove toxins from the body. As an anti-inflammatory, it is rich in B vitamins providing nervous system support and aiding the body in coping with stress. It also contains high level of minerals such as magnesium which helps to relax the muscles, prevent migraines, and has also been shown to have positive effects on reducing depression.

Uses – I often add buckwheat to salads and regularly use buckwheat pasta but it also works well for making noodles, bread and pancakes.

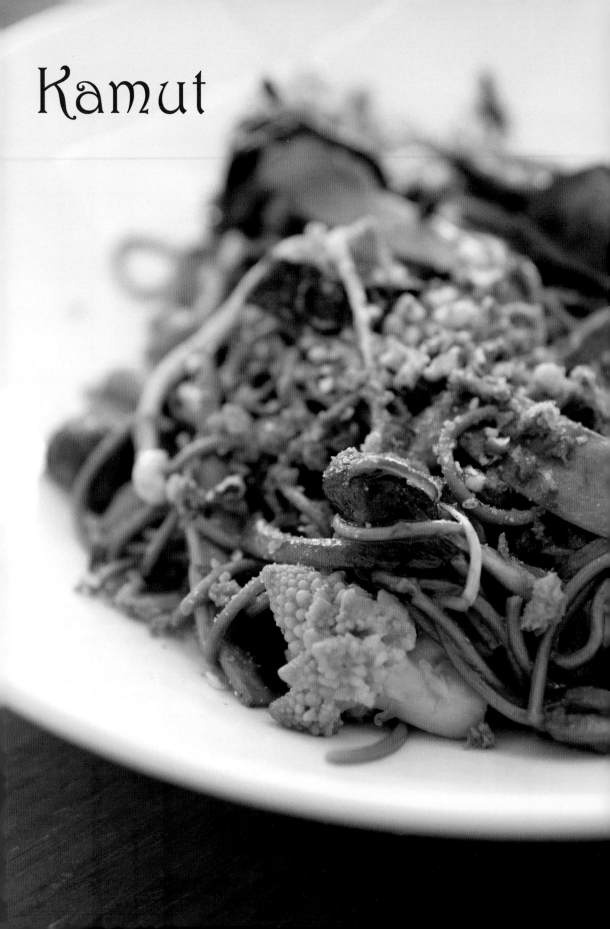

Kamut

Kamut Vegan Noodles

Ingredients

1 cup water (you can add eggs in place of the water if you want to add more bite to your noodles)

1 tablespoon apple cider vinegar
3 cups kamut flour

In a large bowl, make a well in the centre of the flour and add the water and vinegar. Using your hands bring the flour in from the edges to combine with the liquid until it forms a stiff dough which may take a couple of minutes. Add a little more water if required.

Place onto the work top and knead for several minutes more until you have smooth dough that is fairly hard. Wrap in cling film and leave to sit at an ambient temperature for at least an hour.

Once it has rested, roll it out to around five millimetre thickness with a rolling pin before cutting into thin strips with a knife or pizza cutter.

Cook in salted boiling water for a couple of minutes, and then serve.

Kamut is a nutritious grain with a nutty, rich flavour that has been popular since ancient times. It has a large kernel and is rich in protein (containing 30 per cent more than wheat), fibre, antioxidants, vitamins B and E as well as iron and magnesium. Containing a high content of niacin (vitamin B3), kamut boosts our endocrine and nervous systems and it also promotes digestive health. As an immune boosting grain, it has been shown to lower cholesterol and prevent damage from free radicals. Researchers have suggested that kamut wheat may reduce the risk of certain cancers and it has also been shown to have positive effects on blood sugar levels too.

Uses – Kamut can be used to make porridge. It makes a great base for salads, delicious granola, and works well in stews. It also works well in stews.

Interesting Fact – Kamut is also known as the pharaoh grain as it was found in the Egyptian tombs.

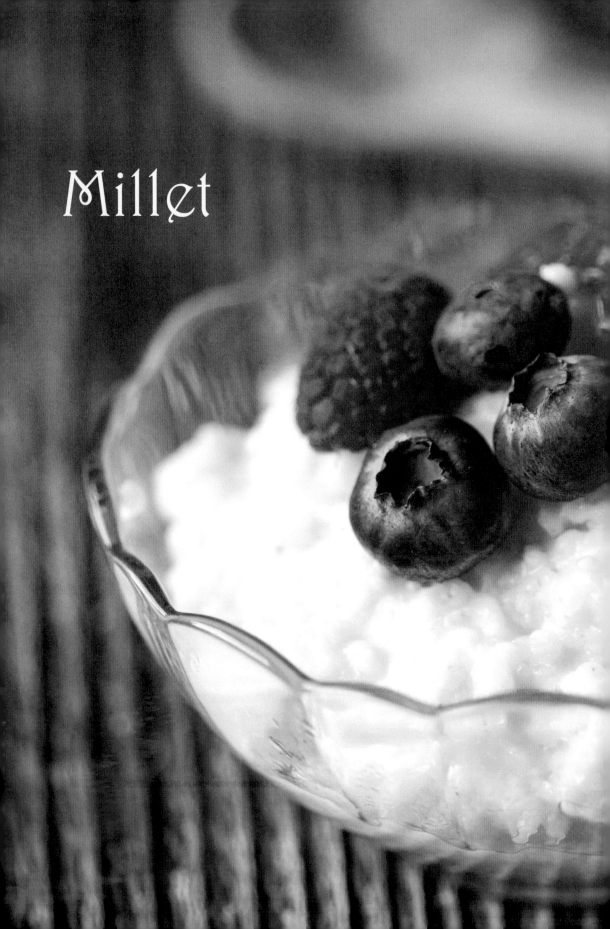

Millet

Cuban Millet

Ingredients

1 carrot chopped
2 cloves garlic minced
1 tablespoon olive oil
1 onion chopped
1 green bell pepper chopped

1 cup of millet
2 cups of vegetable stock
¼ a cup of chopped fresh cilantro
Salt and pepper

Blend the carrot in a food processor until smooth.

Heat the oil in a pan over a medium heat then add the carrot, garlic, pepper and onion and cook for approximately ten minutes until softened.

Add the millet and stir for approximately three minutes until lightly toasted.

Add the vegetable stock, season with salt and pepper before leaving to simmer for 20 minutes until most of the liquid is absorbed and the millet is tender. Stir in the cilantro and it is as simple as that!

Millet is actually the main ingredient in bird seed – but don't let the birds fly off with all the amazing benefits that this super grain has to offer. It is thought to have originated in Africa but it soon became a popular crop in many other parts of the world as it is quick to grow and can tolerate harsh and dry environments. Many developing countries rely on millet to provide basic nutrition. Naturally gluten free, it is rich in B vitamins, magnesium, potassium, zinc, and essential fats. It also contains good levels of protein and fibre. It has been shown to be effective at lowering blood pressure and cholesterol, thus promoting heart health. Millet boosts digestive health and may help to reduce bloating and gas and prevent constipation. Its high magnesium content improves the efficiency of insulin and therefore balances blood sugar levels and may protect against diabetes and it is a fantastic body detoxifier.

Uses – Millet makes a lovely hot cereal and can once again be used in place of rice, pasta or potatoes. It bakes well in muffins and can also be used to make homemade health bars.

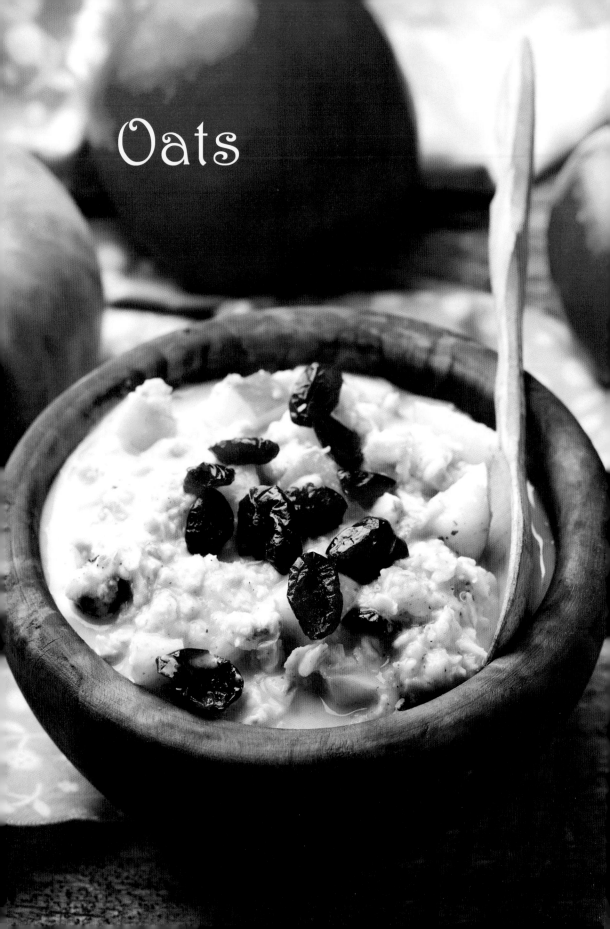

Oats

Overnights Oats with Strawberry and Banana

Ingredients

½ cup of rolled oats

1 cup of coconut milk

1 medium banana chopped

1 cup strawberries chopped

1 tablespoon chia seeds

Combine all the ingredients and place in the fridge overnight. By morning you will have the most delicious readymade breakfast.

Oats are often overlooked for more fashionable so called health foods, but make no mistake, they have earned their place in my list of super grains. Adding oats to your diet on a regular basis can provide a wide range of health benefits. Probably the most well-known is their ability to help lower cholesterol and promote a healthy heart. Being a fantastic source of soluble fibre, this affects the cholesterol levels as it breaks down as it passes through the digestive tract, leaving a gel like substance which then traps substances such as cholesterol containing bile acids, thus reducing the amount of cholesterol that is absorbed into the bloodstream. But the benefits of oats don't stop there! Oats have also been shown to be effective in reducing blood pressure, keeping bowel movements regular and promoting a healthy digestive system as well as reducing the risk of cancer due to their content of natural compounds called phytochemicals.

Famed for being the perfect breakfast for athletes, oats have been shown to improve metabolism and performance when they are eaten an hour before exercise. They can also aid weight loss as part of a healthy diet, keeping you feeling fuller for longer. New research has even shown that children between the ages of two and eighteen who eat oats regularly are 50 per cent less likely to become overweight. Containing amino acids, essential fatty acids and essential vitamins and minerals, oats are an all-round health boosting food.

Uses – Don't save your oats simply for your morning porridge, as they can also be used to make delicious homemade granolas, crunchy toppings for chicken or fish and delicious oat muffins or cookies. My son has his own super flapjack recipe which he makes himself and it really is delicious!

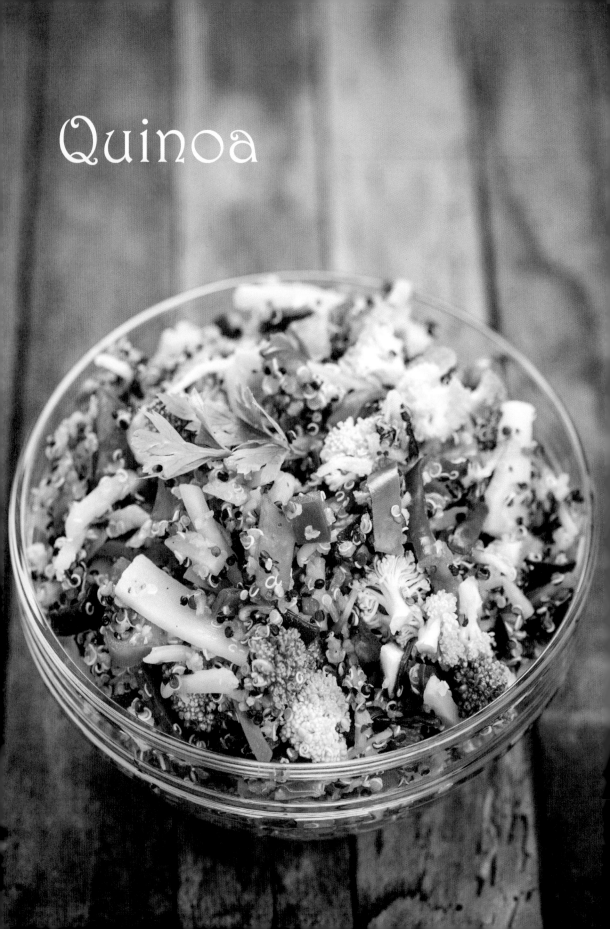

Quinoa

Super Quick Quinoa and Black Beans

Ingredients

1 cup cooked quinoa
1/3 cup of canned black beans
   drained and rinsed
1 small tomato chopped

1 scallion sliced
1 teaspoon of lemon juice
1 teaspoon of olive oil
Salt and pepper to season

Simply combine all the ingredients and serve. This makes a great on the go lunch.

Although considered a grain, quinoa is actually a relative of green, leafy vegetables, as it is derived from the quinoa plant which is related to spinach. Containing more vitamins, nutrients and antioxidants than any other grain, quinoa has become extremely popular, being available in most supermarkets and apprearing on many menus. It is gluten free and high in protein and one of the few plant foods to contain all nine essential amino acids. Quinoa is rich in flavonoids which have been shown to have antiviral, anti-inflammatory and anti-cancer effects. It has more than twice the amount of fibre than most other grains although when boiled it contains less as it absorbs so much water. High in iron, magnesium, potassium and zinc, it is also proven to have a positive effect on blood sugar levels. A good addition to anyone wanting to reduce their weight and calorie intake as the high protein content boosts the metabolism and reduces appetite and the fibre keeps you feeling fuller for longer.

Uses – There are three types of quinoa – red, white and black. We use quinoa flakes for porridge and as a replacement for rice or pasta. It can be used to make delicious salads, and it works brilliantly as a stuffing for mushrooms, peppers or tomatoes and it also makes a fantastic crust for meat or fish. If you haven't already joined the quinoa fan club then I suggest you sign up now.

Interesting Fact – NASA scientists have been looking at it as a suitable crop to be grown in space due to how easy it is to grow, use and how nutritious it is.

Rye

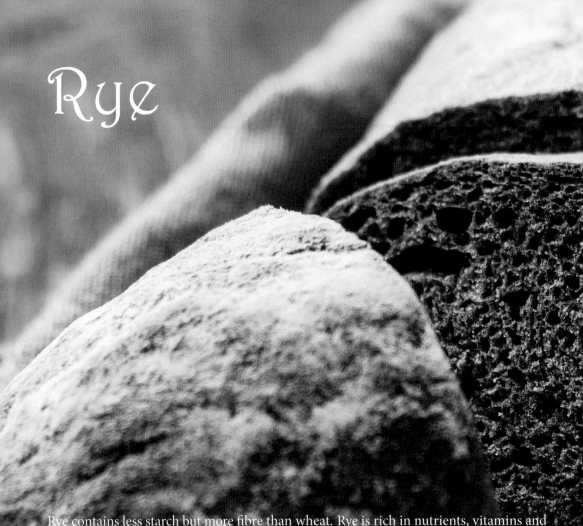

Rye contains less starch but more fibre than wheat. Rye is rich in nutrients, vitamins and minerals, and is an excellent source of fibre, magnesium, phosphorous, manganese and copper. The type of fibre contained in rye is effective in binding with water molecules and therefore maintains a feeling of fullness for much longer. Composed of larger molecules, rye takes longer to break down and does not affect blood sugar levels. A super heart healthy grain, it has been shown to be effective in reducing blood pressure as well as cutting the risk of gallstones too. It is fantastic for the digestive system and intestines and as with many of the super grains, it may be linked to the prevention of certain cancers.

Uses – I am certain everyone will have tried delicious rye bread at some point which is now readily available but don't stop there – rye cookies, pancakes, waffles, pasta and crackers are all super delicious too.

Interesting Fact – Our ancestors in Northern and Eastern Europe used rye bread to provide energy for hard and physical work. Rye remains one of the top five consumed grains on the planet.

Black Rye Bread

Ingredients

2¼ teaspoons of active dry yeast

320-400ml warm water

1 teaspoon brown sugar

2 tablespoons cocoa powder

2 tablespoons ground espresso beans

70ml molasses

3 teaspoons of caraway seeds plus extra for garnish

3 tablespoons of unsalted butter cubed

150g grated carrot

150g rye flour

2 teaspoons sea salt

425g bread flour plus a little extra for dusting

A little olive oil

A little milk

Whisk the yeast with 320ml of the warm water and the sugar and set aside until it is creamy and foamy.

Place a small saucepan on a medium heat and add the cocoa, coffee, molasses, caraway, butter and salt and stir until melted.

In a large bowl, mix the yeast mixture with the molasses mixture and add the carrot.

Add the flours and stir until you have a sticky dough. If your dough is too dry add a little more of the warm water. Alternatively, if the dough is too wet, add a little more flour.

Place the dough on the worktop and knead for five minutes until it is springy and elastic. Shape into a ball, rub with olive oil and place the seam side down in an oiled bowl. Cover and place somewhere warm for one to two hours until the dough has risen by at least one half.

Using your fist, press down on the dough, flattening it a little. Remove from the bowl and reshape it into a ball, and once again, rub with the olive oil, place seam side down in an oiled baking tray, cover and leave somewhere warm until it has doubled in size, probably leaving it for one more hour.

Uncover, brush with a little milk, dust with a little flour and sprinkle with the remaining caraway seeds. Bake for 20 minutes at 220°C before reducing the heat to 180°C and baking for a further 25 minutes until the loaf has a lovely crust and makes a hollow sound when tapped on the base.

Allow to cool for 15 minutes prior to serving.

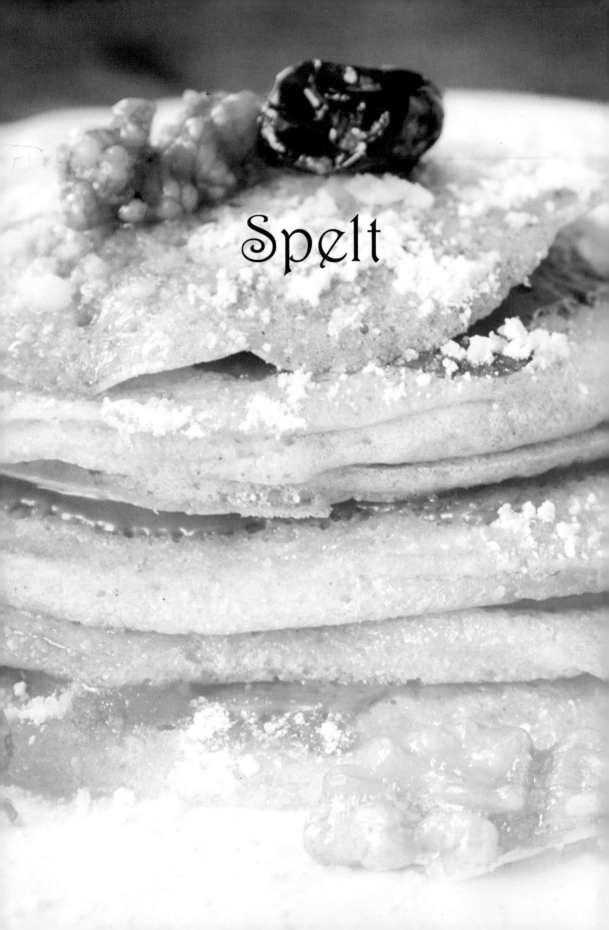

Spelt

Healthy Spelt Pancakes

Ingredients

½ a cup of spelt flour

½ a teaspoon cinnamon

Pinch of salt

1 teaspoon baking powder

¼ teaspoon maca powder

½ a tablespoon of vegan protein
powder

½ a cup of almond or soya milk

Chia seeds, coconut shavings, cacao nibs, goji berries and almond butter for topping

Mix all the dry ingredients together then add the milk and mix well. Add a little oil to a pan on medium heat and spoon the mixture into the pan.

Cook on both sides then serve with your choice of toppings.

Spelt has definitely gained in popularity over recent years, and just last week I noticed that my supermarket now stocks spelt pizza bases and spelt pasta – spelt bread has long been readily available. It is suggested that spelt is not only more nutrient dense that wheat but more flavoursome too with its distinctly nutty taste.

Particularly high in phosphorous and protein which are necessary for the growth and development of new tissues, bones, organs, blood vessels and muscles as well as new cells, spelt is an excellent source of thiamine (a B vitamin) which helps to boost the immune system. Unusually for a grain, it is rich in B vitamins which help the body to cope with stress and to promote a healthy nervous system.

Spelt is rich in fibre too, promoting good digestive health and preventing constipation, bloating and gas and aiding the reduction of cholesterol. It contains many bone boosting vitamins and minerals as well as riboflavin which studies have shown can prevent migraine attacks. This super grain promotes a healthy heart and may reduce the risk of gallstones.

Uses – So how can you incorporate it into your daily diet? The answer is very easily. Spelt noodles, cookies, scones, pizza dough and pancakes are all delicious.

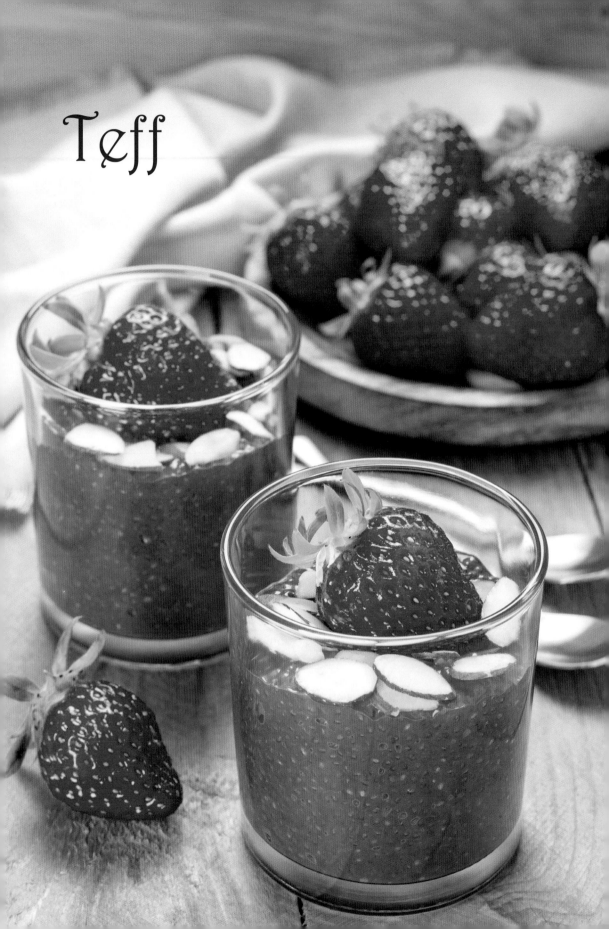

Teff

Teff Crumbled Apples

Ingredients

4 large apples thinly sliced
½ teaspoon cinnamon

Pinch of sea salty
1 cup apple juice

For the crumble:
1½ cups of rolled oats
½ a cup of teff flour
¼ of a cup maple syrup or rice
  syrup

¼ cup of canola oil
½ teaspoon of cinnamon
Sea salt

Preheat the oven to 175°C and place the apples into an ovenproof dish.

Sprinkle with cinnamon and salt and pour over the apple juice. Mix together all the crumble ingredients and pour over the apples.

Bake for 30 minutes until the crumble is golden and crisp and the apples are tender. The smell of cinnamon will fill your whole house – yummy! This also works well with pears and pear juice.

Teff is a fine grain only the size of a poppy seed that comes in a range of colours. It grows mainly in Ethiopia and has a mild, nutty flavour. It is possible to buy teff whole, and to cook it the same way you would cook quinoa or in the form of flour which makes a wonderful addition to many baking recipes. Naturally gluten free and bursting with fibre, it is rich in protein and calcium, making it a bone boosting grain and also an excellent source of iron. `

Uses – Teff is fabulous when used for baking in cookies, breads, brownies, and it makes a delicious chocolate pudding, pancakes, porridge and even pastries!

Interesting Fact – The word teff actually translates as 'lost' probably referring to the minute size of the grains.

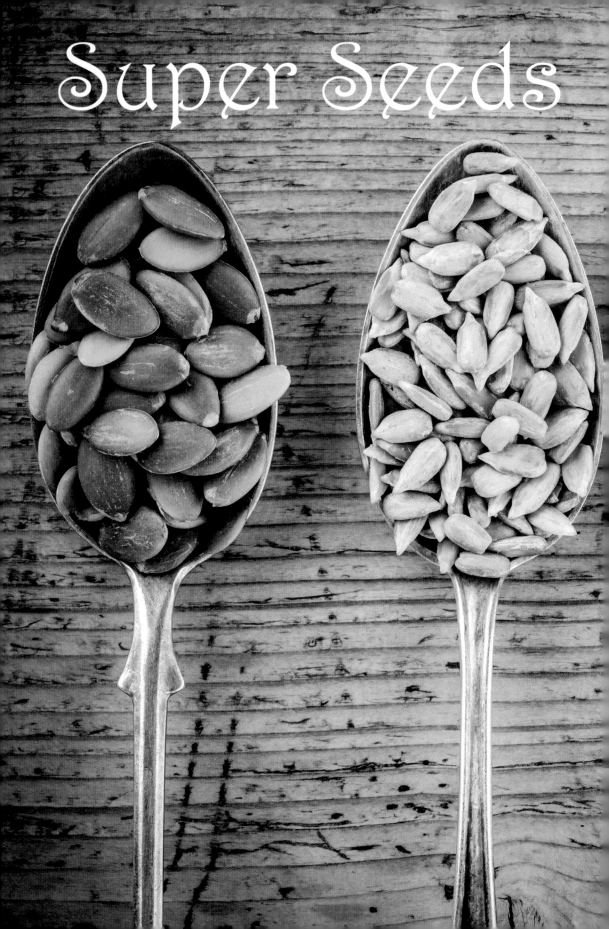

Super Seeds

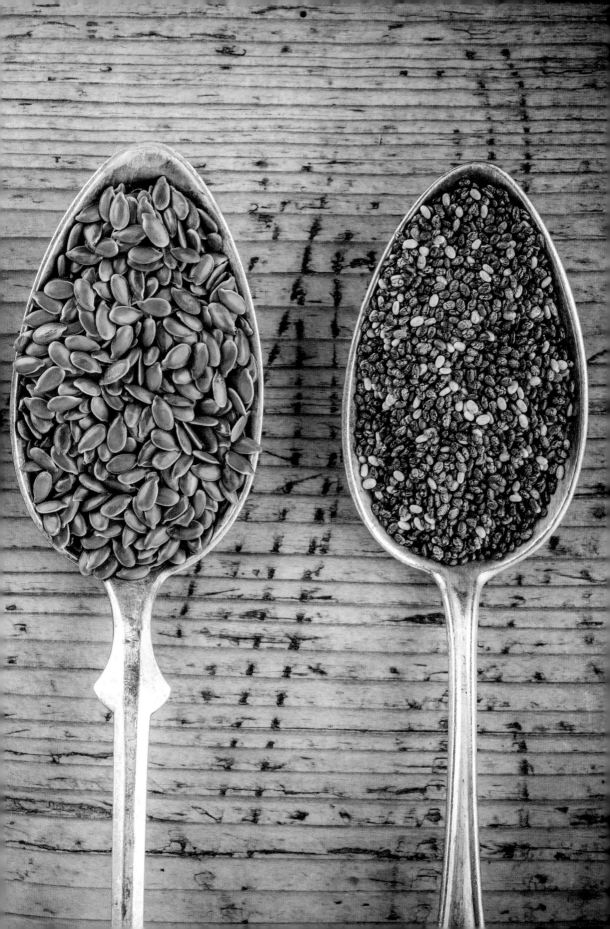

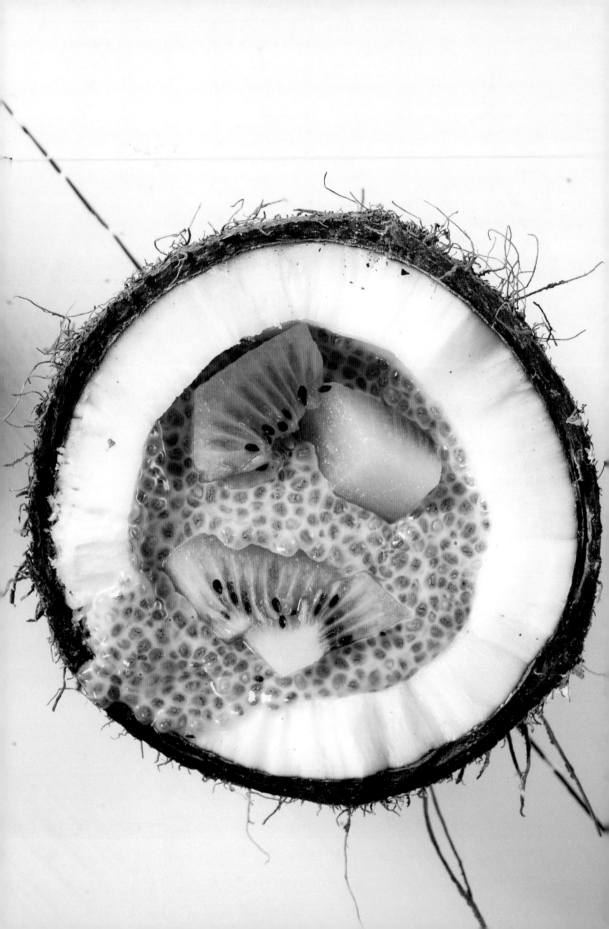

Have I mentioned already how much I love seeds? These tiny powerhouses of nutrition are so versatile and delicious. Not a day goes by that I don't add seeds to my diet in one form or another, and my whole family loves them too. Always my go to snack, I always have a bag of seeds in my handbag in case I get hungry between meals. Despite their miniscule size, seeds are filled with super high concentrations of vitamins, minerals, proteins and healthy oils. So it is time for you to start incorporating them into your daily diet too; a good start would be my favourite super seeds.

Apricot Seeds

Apricot kernels are the seed of the fruit of the apricot tree. Originating in Armenia and Northern China, they are now readily available whole or pre-dried. These nutritious seeds are responsible for the almond flavour in several liqueurs, amaretto cookies and marzipan, and they are also a common ingredient in massage oils. Apricot seeds are either bitter or sweet, and most people prefer the sweet variety as they have a milder taste. The bitter kernels have actually been used in Chinese medicine for many years to treat a wide range of conditions, such as respiratory illnesses including colds and asthma. Eaten on a regular basis, both kinds can promote a strong immune system better equipped to resist infections.

Marzipan

Ingredients

1¼ cup of almonds unblanched and unroasted

2 tablespoons apricot seeds ground

2¼ cups of dark brown sugar

3 egg whites

Place the almonds, seeds and sugar in a blender and blend until you have a very fine powder.

Pour the powder into a bowl then one at a time with your fingers, knead in the egg whites and continue kneading the mixture until it is smooth and elastic. It may be formed into shapes or simply rolled out – either way it will be delicious!

Apricot seeds are rich in vitamin B17, which is excellent for regulating blood pressure levels, and being healthy fats helps to support heart health and reduce cholesterol. Apricot seeds are also a natural anti-inflammatory, as they have been shown to relieve pain and the symptoms of arthritis. Thought to be a natural laxative too, they may be effective in treating constipation and maintaining regular bowel movements.

Uses – Of course there is homemade marzipan, and the bitter sweet taste of the kernels makes a delicious chocolate butter which is good to eat straight from the jar. They can be added to homemade granola or soaked with oats overnight for a delicious bircher muesli. They also work well in spicy rice dishes, and the ground powder can be used in baking or even to make homemade energy and snack bars. **Apricot Kernels contain a substance that when consumed in very high doses may be toxic so take advice from your doctor if you are pregnant.**

Interesting Fact – Did you know that apricot kernels have long been thought to be an aphrodisiac? Even William Shakespeare wrote about them as such!

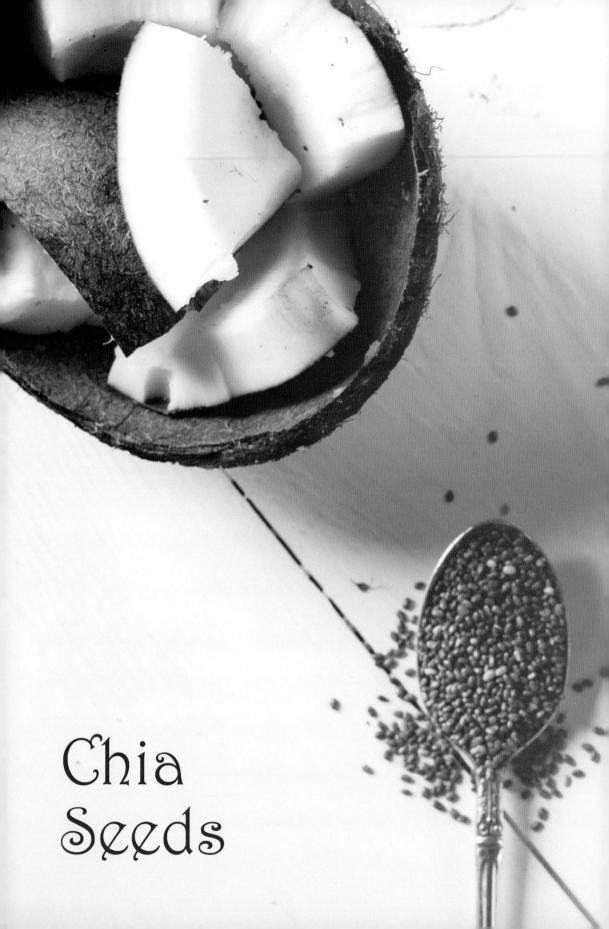

Chia
Seeds

Chia Coconut Pudding

Ingredients

2 tablespoons chia seeds   1 cup water
1 tablespoon coconut milk powder   Honey to taste

Grind the chia seeds – I find a coffee grinder works best for this, or you can use a blender with a grinder attachment.

Pour the water into a pan and add the coconut milk powder and bring to the boil. Remove from the heat. (If you want this to be a cold pudding omit the heating step).

Whisk in the chia seeds. Leave for a couple of minutes then whisk again.

Pour into serving glasses. Leave to stand further until the pudding has thickened further before drizzling with honey and serving. This is also lovely with berries on the top.

Chia seeds contain 10 times more fibre than rice; three times more antioxidants than blueberries; three times more iron than spinach; six times more calcium than milk; eight times more Omega-3 than salmon; eight times more vitamin C than oranges; twice the potassium of a banana, and 15 times more magnesium than broccoli.

Full of vitamins, minerals, fibre, protein and antioxidants, chia seeds may aid with the reduction of joint pain, weight loss, boost heart health and brain function, improve depression and symptoms associated with arthritis as well as protecting the liver. Naturally gluten free, they are a great detoxifier and can help to reduce blood pressure and aid with weight loss.

Uses – I know you are eager to add them into your diet so here is how you can – chia seeds actually make a fantastic egg replacement in recipes, soak in water or milk overnight to make the perfect base for breakfast in the morning, mix into muffin mix, add to cereals or granola, add to yoghurt and fruit or use as a healthy coating for fish, meat or vegetables.

Interesting Fact – Chia seeds are the richest plant source of Omega-3 fatty acids and chia comes from the Mayan word meaning 'strength'.

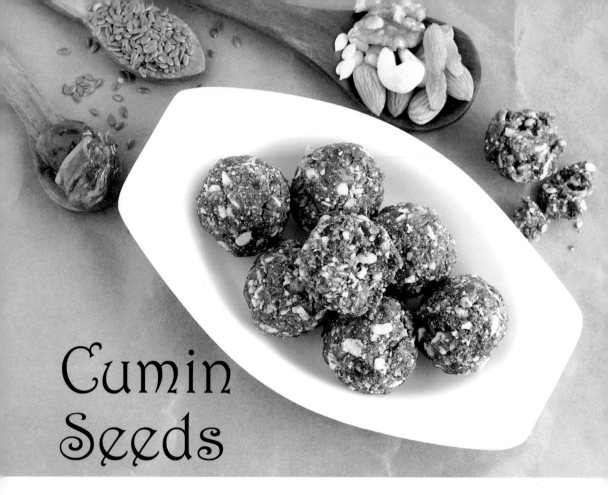

Cumin Seeds

Cumin is a small flowering plant, native to the Middle East although today it is grown all over the world. This plant produces small, greyish yellow seeds with ridges which are very well known for their distinctive spicy flavour, although probably much less well known for their amazing health benefits. Not only are these seeds a fantastic source of minerals such as magnesium, zinc, iron, copper, potassium, calcium and selenium, but they are also rich in aromatic essential oils. The copper and iron content boosts red blood cell production and formation and gives the liver a boost too; magnesium relaxes the muscles and aids blood flow; potassium regulates body fluids and may promote a healthy blood pressure; zinc boosts the immune system and collagen production and the calcium and magnesium combination make these seeds a bone boosting addition to our diets.

Cumin seeds are also rich in antioxidants, phytochemicals and fibre and have been proven to aid digestion and maintain healthy movement in our intestines thus preventing constipation. Full of vitamins A, C, E and B vitamins, their antibacterial, antifungal and anti-inflammatory properties have also made cumin a common asthma remedy. Cumin seeds are also an excellent source of melatonin which if taken before bed may prevent insomnia and promote restful sleep. For optimum effect, mix with a ripe banana. It is possible to buy both cumin seeds or powder although I always recommend the powder as it contains the highest concentration of good quality nutrients. Also, once ground which can be done by hand with a pestle and mortar or with a coffee mill, it is best stored in the fridge and used quickly as its flavour will start to fade.

Moroccan Vegetable Stew

Ingredients

2 tablespoons olive oil

3 cloves garlic crushed

1 teaspoon ground coriander

1 teaspoon ground cumin

½ teaspoon ground cayenne

¼ teaspoon ground cinnamon

5 cups of vegetable stock

4 carrots peeled and cut into chunks

2½ cups of peeled aubergine diced

2½ cups of courgette sliced

2 cups of cauliflower florets

1 cup of onion diced

1 can (15oz) chickpeas drained and rinsed

2 cans of chopped tomatoes

¾ cup of dried currants

1 cup of toasted almond flakes

½ tablespoon kosher salt

Heat the oil in a pan and add the garlic and spices and cook on a medium heat stirring for around two minutes.

Place this mixture into a slow cooker. Add the vegetable stock, aubergine, courgette, onion, carrots, cauliflower, chickpeas, currants, almonds and salt and stir well.

Cook slowly for eight to nine hours on high until the vegetables are tender.

Take three ladles of the mixture and place in a blender and blend until smooth before returning it to the rest of the mixture and stirring well.

Ladle into bowls and serve with quinoa and a small side salad.

Uses – They are a good addition to a wide range of dishes from Mediterranean, to Asian, and Chinese to Indian. Fantastic with meat, fish, rice and vegetable dishes, they are also great in soups and sauces. Have a go at cumin curried potatoes or rub cumin onto pork and roast, give a kick both of flavour and nutrients to vegan burgers and if you haven't tried black bean soup then you are seriously missing out. Curried cauliflower is a healthy alternative to cauliflower cheese or you could just stick with the well-known chicken tikka masala – the possibilities are endless so have fun with it!

Interesting Fact – Cumin is often used to treat the symptoms of the common cold and some people drink cumin juice as a general all round health tonic although this is not something I have tried myself.

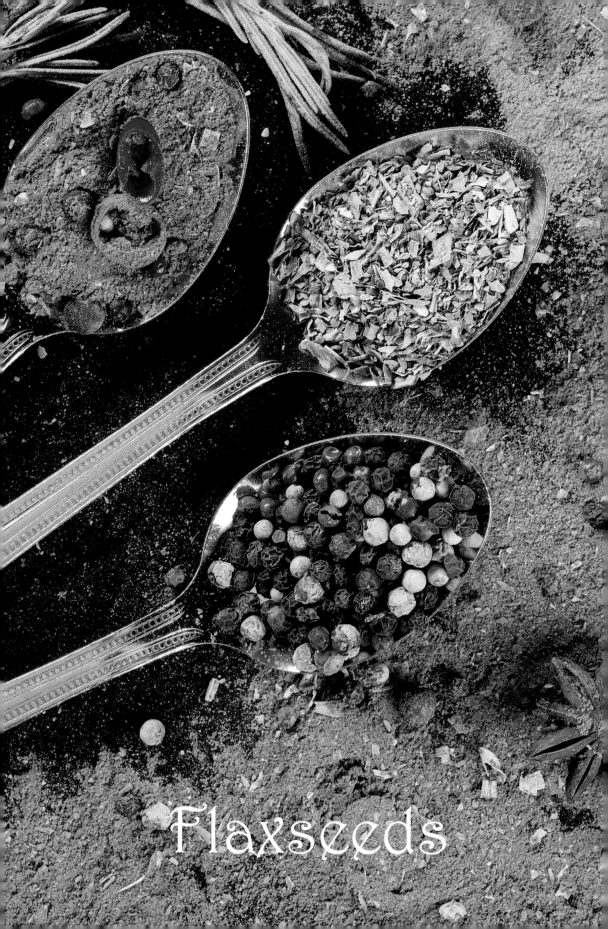

Flaxseeds

Crusted Salmon Fillets

Ingredients

4 salmon fillets

4 tablespoons milled flaxseeds

4 tablespoons freshly squeezed
  lemon juice

4 teaspoons coconut oil

1 teaspoon cracked black pepper

Preheat the oven to 180°C.

Mix the flaxseeds, coconut oil, lemon juice and pepper together in a bowl to make a paste.

Place the salmon fillets onto a lined baking tray then spread the paste evenly over the four fillets.

Bake in the oven for 15 to 20 minutes until the salmon is cooked and the crust is perfectly crisp and browned. Serve the fish over charred asparagus.

The main health benefits of flaxseeds come from their rich content of alpha linolenic acid (a powerful anti-inflammatory), fibre and lignans, which are plant compounds that have oestrogen like effects and antioxidant properties, thus reducing symptoms of the menopause and regulating hormones as well as possibly reducing the risk of breast and prostate cancers. Bursting with fibre, one tablespoon of flaxseeds provides more fibre than half a cup of oat bran.

Uses – I love to put them in my smoothies, although ground flaxseeds can be added to virtually any meal from soups, salads, stir fries, and casseroles, or they can be used to make a nutritious crust for meat or fish.

Important tip – To obtain maximum benefits, flaxseeds should be consumed milled. When I buy them whole, I put them in a coffee grinder then store them in a fridge to maintain freshness although they are readily available pre-ground. If not ground down you will very often see them pass straight through whole!

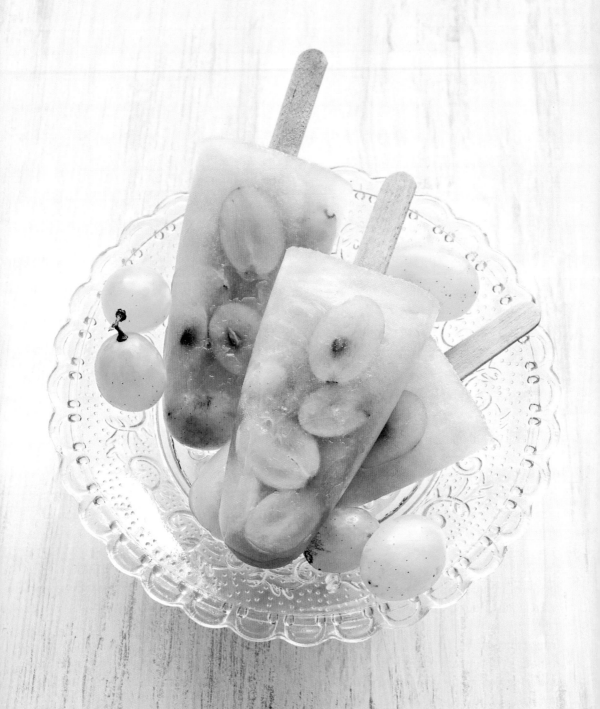

Grape Seeds

Frosted Grapes

So quick and simple yet utterly delicious and super cool (in appearance and temperature!).

Ingredients
2 cups of seeded grapes washed

Place into an air tight bag and freeze overnight – how easy is that?

Whilst grapes are one of the most popular fruits appearing in most fruit bowls and every lunch box, most people avoid eating what is probably the most nutritious part – the seeds! So where do their powerful health benefits stem from? Well they are SUPER rich in antioxidants and plant compounds known as oligomeric proanthocyanidin complexes or OPCs. They not only resist the damaging free radicals preventing premature ageing and the development of many diseases but according to the *Journal of Alternative Medicine Review* OPCs may even play a role in cancer prevention. Research has shown that grape seeds improve circulation and improve flexibility in joints and tissues. They have been linked to a reduction in cognitive decline as well as preventing cavities and reversing tooth decay. They have also been shown to improve bone strength and to reduce blood pressure.

Now we have all been guilty of selecting the seedless grapes in the supermarket, but from now on opt for the seeded varieties. However, to get the maximum benefit, you would have to eat a lot of grapes but luckily you can buy grape seeds – although they are a little bitter, or grape seed extract which is extremely popular. Grape seed extract is actually ground up seeds and a general dosage would be 150-350mg daily although up to 600mg can be taken daily with no known side effects.

Uses – As for the grape seeds themselves, grapes containing seeds work well in so many different recipes. You can make a delicious Waldorf salad, add them to your morning or post workout smoothie, slice and add to freshly made juice pops – these look amazing by the way and are always a visual hit with both children and adults. Grapes also work well with peanut butter so maybe try these in a wrap or for a real twist try roasting grapes, with walnuts and olives with a little thyme – just delicious.

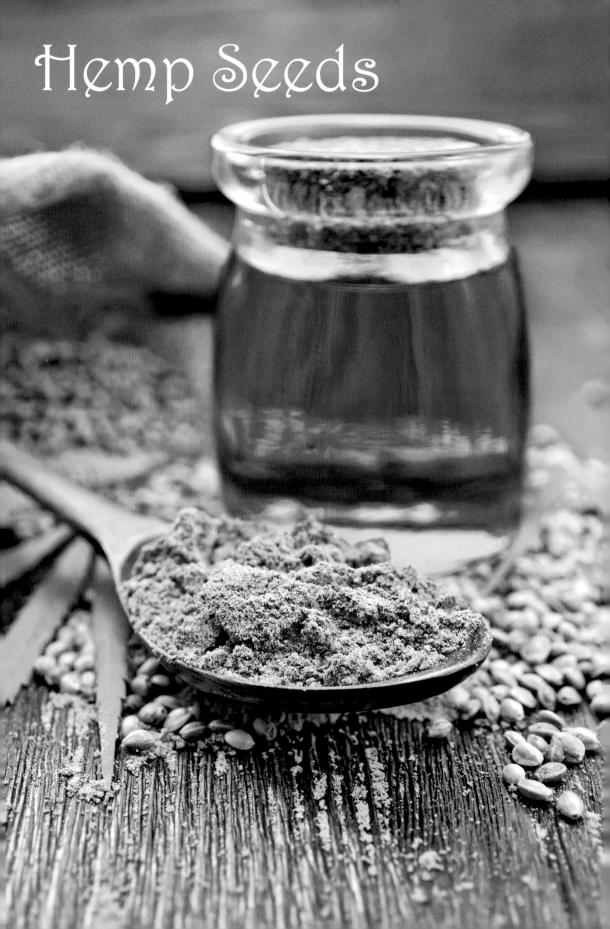

Hemp Seeds

Lentil Hemp Burgers

Ingredients

2 cups lentils rinsed, boiled and
  drained

¼ onion chopped

2 cloves of garlic minced

½ teaspoon of dried rosemary

½ teaspoon of dried sage

½ teaspoon of dried oregano

1 tablespoon hemp flour

½ cup of rolled oats

1 cup of hulled hemp seeds

1 egg

Salt and pepper to season and oil
  for cooking

Place all the ingredients into a food processor and blend.

Take handfuls of the mixture, shape into patties and place onto a lined baking tray. Chill for at least one hour.

Heat a little oil in a pan and add the patties, cooking for approximately three minutes on each side until hot and golden. Serve on a bun with salad and a little guacamole.

Hemp seeds contain all 20 amino acids including the nine essential amino acids that our bodies cannot produce and they contain a perfect three to one ratio of Omega-6 and Omega-3 fatty acids, promoting a healthy heart and immune system. In fact, these essential fatty acids may reduce cholesterol, blood pressure, heart disease and stroke. They have a concentrated balance of proteins, fats, vitamins, minerals and enzymes and are one of the world's most healthy foods. They are a more digestible form of protein than meat, eggs, cheese or milk, and hemp oil contains more Omega-3 than any fish or fish oil supplement. Hemp has been shown to improve circulation and reduce inflammation, it is therefore beneficial to arthritis sufferers.

An effective energy and immune booster, bursting with B vitamins and vitamins E and D as well as fibre, calcium, magnesium, copper, potassium and phosphorous, hemp seeds have been said to aid, if not heal, sufferers of immune deficiency diseases.

Uses – They can be used to make delicious hemp milk; and they can be added to salads, smoothies and cereals. Add to mashed potato for a flavour boost or sprinkle them on yoghurts or porridge, grind them to make a delicious hemp seed butter or use hemp four in baking.

Pomegranate Seeds

Kale Salad with Pomegranate and Walnuts

Ingredients

1 bunch of kale washed and torn
2 tablespoons of olive oil
1 tablespoon fresh lime juice
½ teaspoon freshly grated ginger
½ a cup pomegranate seeds

2 tablespoons chopped red onion
¼ of a cup of toasted and chopped
  walnuts
Sea salt and cracked black pepper

Rub the kale with the olive oil, lime and ginger until completely coated then place in a large salad bowl. Add the pomegranate seeds, red onion and walnuts and toss. Season with the salt and pepper.

Pomegranates are super high in polyphenols, a form of antioxidant linked to reducing the risk of cancer and heart disease. Rich in vitamin C, fibre, antioxidants and anti-inflammatories, the health benefits of pomegranate seeds are well worth the time and effort it takes to break through the skin and uncover the slimy cased seeds inside. Native to Iran and traced back to as early as 3000BC, pomegranate seeds are rich in potassium and help to reduce blood pressure. They are high in fibre, so aid a healthy digestive system and helping to curb hunger, and just one portion contains over 40 per cent of our daily recommended amount of vitamin C.

Various studies have shown that drinking pomegranate juice can prevent the formation of plaque. It has been linked to improved metal agility and a reduced risk of Alzheimer's disease due to a polyphenal called punicalagin, which increases the level of oxygen in the blood, allowing it to flow freely and prevent blood clots. It is also shown to prevent the hardening of the artery walls as well as reducing the damage to cartilage caused by arthritis.

Uses – Simply delicious added to porridge or muesli, a bright addition to any salad, try making pomegranate jam or add to smoothies.

Interesting Fact – Pomegranate juice is said to have more health boosting properties than green tea and red wine.

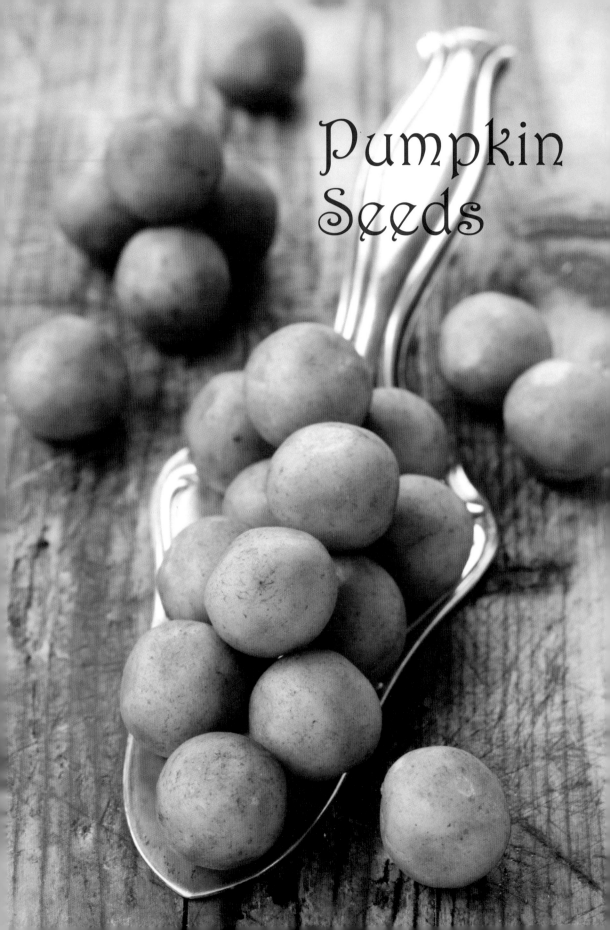

Pumpkin
Seeds

Fiery Pumpkin Seeds

Ingredients

1 cup fresh pumpkin seeds
2 teaspoons hot sauce
1 teaspoon chilli powder
½ teaspoon salt

½ teaspoon ground cumin
¼ teaspoon cayenne pepper
¼ teaspoon pepper

Mix the pumpkin seeds with the hot sauce.

In a bowl, combine the chilli powder, cumin, cayenne pepper, pepper and salt. Pour this mix into the bowl with the pumpkin seeds and ensure they are all coated.

Spread the seeds onto a lined baking sheet and place in a preheated oven for 45 to 50 minutes, stirring occasionally until the seeds are crisp and dry. Allow to cool then store in an airtight jar.

Super rich in protein, with just 10g providing 54 per cent of your daily requirement, pumpkin seeds are also rich in B vitamins as well as that mood boosting and calming tryptophan, an amino acid that produces serotonin. Pumpkin seeds are also famed for preventing kidney stones as well as parasites. Rich in immune-boosting zinc, which is also good for bone health, they are also natural antioxidants as well as being antifungal and antiviral. They may protect against certain types of cancer and diabetes. So next time you are carving that pumpkin, DO NOT throw away the scooped out insides as that really is the treasure.

Uses – There are so many uses for pumpkin seeds either as a snack or added to cereals and muesli; for a lovely topping to homemade bread, or scattered on top of a bowl of hot soup, added to cookies, health bars or granola – the list is endless.

Interesting Fact – Pumpkin seeds are the only alkaline forming seeds.

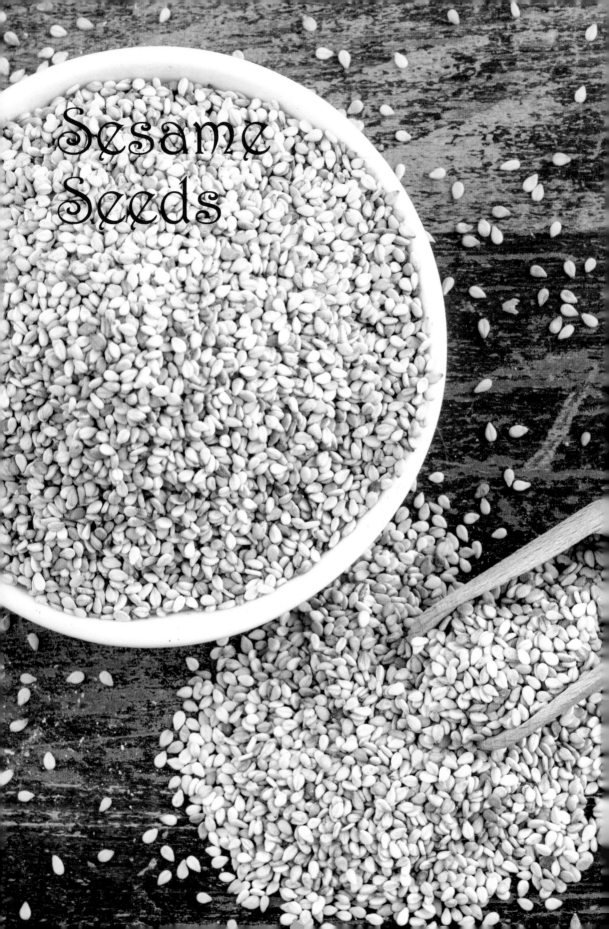

Sesame
Seeds

Sesame Seed Prune Balls

Ingredients

½ a cup raw cashew nuts
½ a cup of pumpkin seeds
1 cup raw tahini
1 cup of prunes

½ teaspoon vanilla extract
½ cup sesame seeds
2/3 cup of dried shredded coconut

Place all the ingredients except the sesame seeds into a food processor and grind the mixture until it forms a thick paste.

Place the sesame seeds into a bowl.

Take tablespoons of the mixture and roll into a ball between the palms of your hands then roll the balls into the sesame seeds until fully covered. Place onto a lined tray. Repeat until all the mixture has been made into balls.

Place into the freezer for around 30 minutes to chill and firm up. These can be stored in an airtight container for up to a week.

Sesame seeds are famous for their super oil which is resistant to rancidity. This oil has been linked to preventing diabetes and lowering blood pressure. Sesame seeds contain phytosterols which block the production of cholesterol and their high zinc content boosts collagen production, promoting healthy hair, skin, nails and joints and also boosting the immune system. Rich in calcium and magnesium, so bone boosting, these minerals coupled with thiamine and tryptophan make sesame seeds a true stress reliever and may promote restful sleep. They have been shown to prevent and relieve arthritis and even protect the liver from the harmful effects of alcohol. Black sesame seeds are rich in iron so good for preventing anaemia and sesame seed oil has been shown to promote hair health.

Uses – If you have never tried tahini then you are seriously missing out, sesame seeds work wonderfully with Asian flavours so try sticky sesame chicken, add to salads or soups and sprinkle over cooked vegetables to add a delicious health boost.

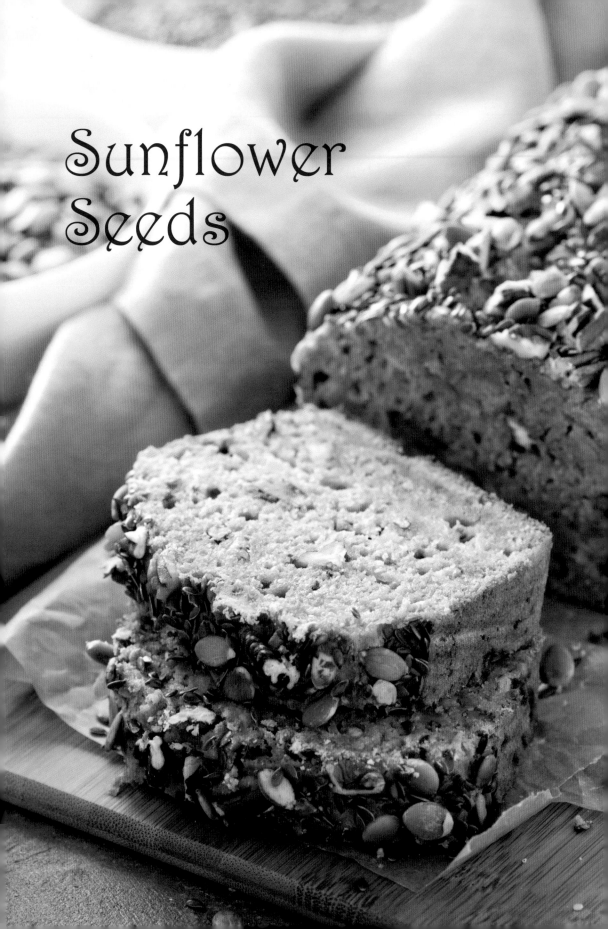

Sunflower Seeds

Sunflower Seed Buttercups

Ingredients

½ cup of sunflower seed butter
2 tablespoons coconut oil
2 tablespoons honey

2 tablespoons dark chocolate chips
  or raw cacao chips
1 tablespoon roasted sunflower
  seeds

Ensure the coconut oil is liquid and at room temperature then mix it with the sunflower seed butter.

Add in the honey and mix well.

Fill a cupcake tray with paper moulds then pour the mixture into the moulds. Sprinkle the top of each mould with toasted sesame seeds and the chocolate chips then freeze for 30 minutes.

It is highly likely I eat sunflower seeds every single day in one form or another. I call them 'happy seeds' as I love the thought that they come from the beautiful large sunflower which turns throughout the day to follow the course of the sun. Originally used 5000 years ago by the native Americans but now we have all caught on to the trend. Sunflower seeds are super rich in vitamin E – this vitamin is excellent for the skin and can protect it from ultraviolet radiation. It is also an antioxidant and prevents cholesterol from oxidizing, which therefore stops it from sticking to the blood vessel walls causing blocked arteries. Vitamin E also has fantastic anti-inflammatory properties and therefore may be effective in reducing the symptoms of arthritis or asthma as well as many other inflammatory related conditions.

These tiny seeds are also an excellent source of copper which encourages the production of collagen and magnesium which promote strong and healthy bones. It is also fantastic at relaxing our muscles and good for muscle recovery after a workout, preventing soreness and fatigue. Sunflower seeds may also be effective in maintaining a healthy blood pressure and has been shown to be effective in preventing migraines. Sunflower seeds also contain tryptophan – the feel good amino acid.

Uses – I think you will struggle not to eat them all straight from the packet but just in case you do need a little more inspiration, sunflower seeds are delicious in bread mixes, cereals, granolas and mueslis, make a lovely topping for soup, can be used in savoury biscuit recipes and I also love adding them to stir fries and rice dishes.

Interesting Fact – Just a quarter of a cup of sunflower seeds provides over 90 per cent of your recommended daily intake of vitamin E.

Take note – Once at room temperature these buttercups (in the above recipe) start to melt very quickly – not that they will last that long anyway!

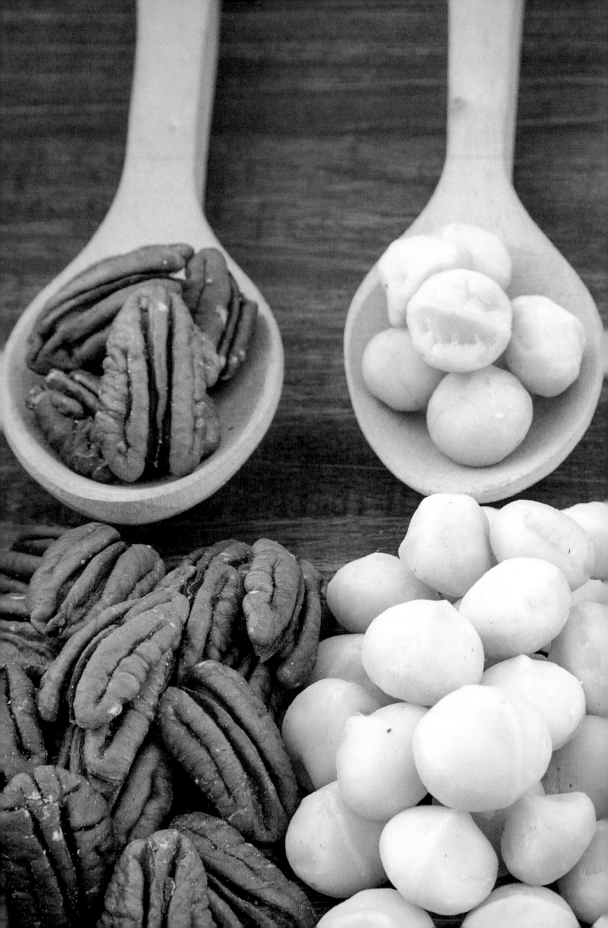

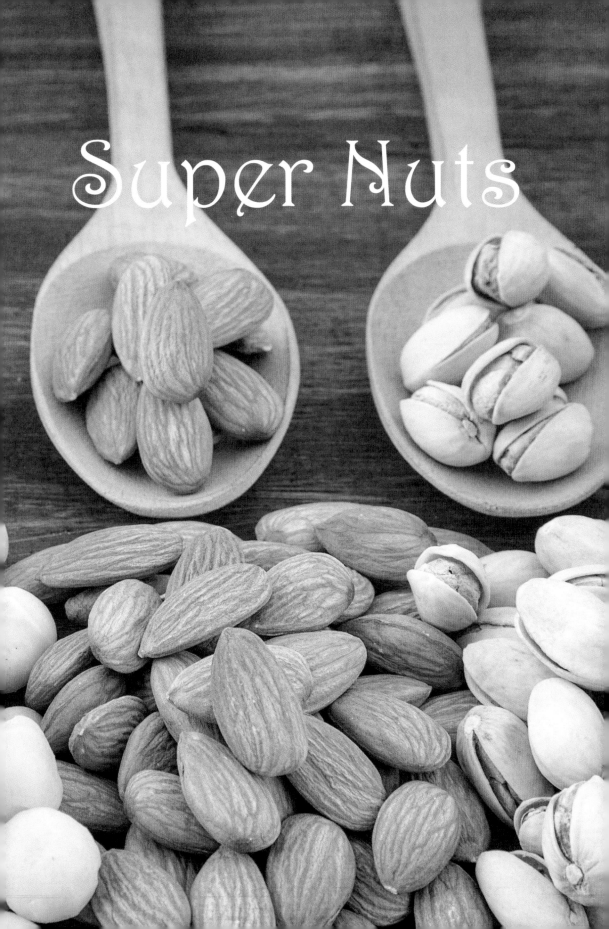

Super Nuts

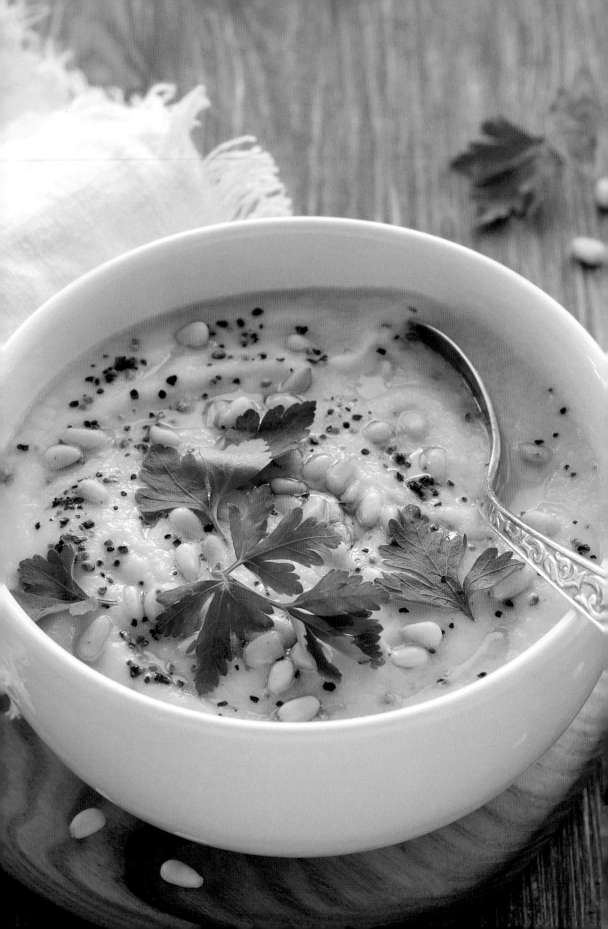

Never ever doubt whether a handful of raw nuts is a super healthy (and delicious and satisfying) snack. People often make the common mistake of simply looking at the calorie or fat content of nuts and discarding them as unhealthy. I can assure you that a 'fat free' diet lacking in essential fats *is* not nutritious, as it could lead to a whole host of health problems. However, some nuts are healthier than others, and my mission is to help you choose the best options. Before we progress, I must point out that peanuts will not make an appearance on my list of super nuts as they are, despite their name, not nuts but legumes. The nuts included in this section are tree nuts whereas peanuts grow underground.

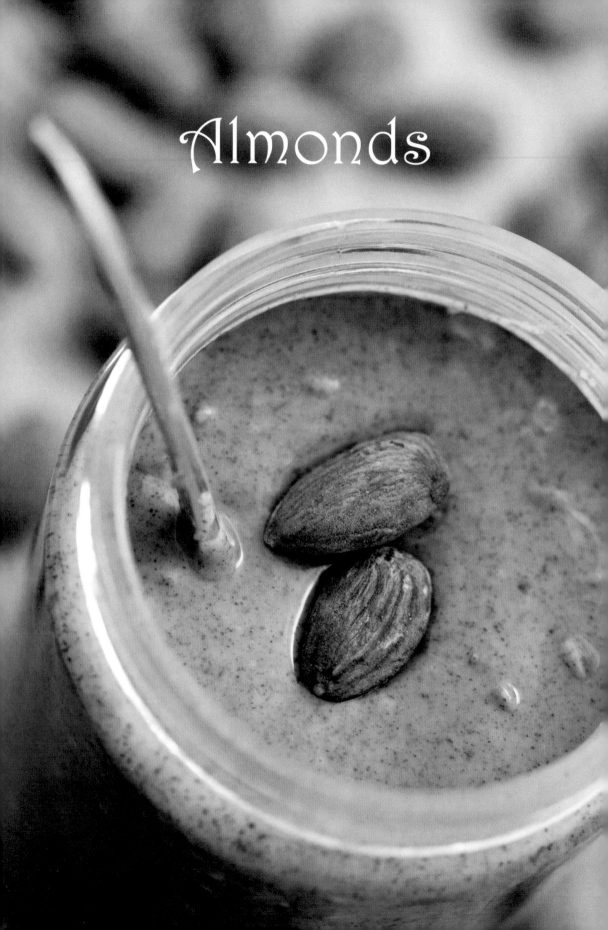

Almonds

Spicy Cauliflower and Almond Soup

Ingredients

1 large onion peeled and chopped

½ cup of raw almonds

1 large cauliflower head cut into florets

1 teaspoon harissa

1 teaspoon cumin

1 litre of chicken or vegetable stock

1 tablespoon of extra virgin olive oil

Salt and pepper for seasoning

Heat the oil in a large pan and add the almonds and onions and cook for a few minutes until the onions are soft.

Add the cauliflower, harissa and cumin and stir for a few more minutes before finally adding the stock.

Bring to the boil then reduce the heat and simmer for 20 minutes. In batches, blend the soup before returning to the pan to return to the perfect temperature for serving.

Serve with a little coriander and freshly baked bread.

Prunus Dulcis is the name given to the almond tree, which is native to the Middle East, although the USA is now the world's largest almond producer. Just one handful of almonds will provide 3.5g of fibre and 6g of protein as well as 37 per cent of your recommended daily requirement of vitamin E, 32 per cent of your recommended daily intake of manganese and 20 per cent of your recommended daily requirement of magnesium. And that's without mentioning all the B vitamins, copper and phosphorous that these nuts are full of. Almonds contain most of their nutrients in their skins. They are rich in antioxidants and a heart healthy nut. In fact, a study in the journal *Circulation* found that people with abnormally high levels of lipids such as cholesterol in the blood were able to significantly reduce their risk factors for coronary heart disease by simply snacking on whole almonds.

Uses – Almonds are delicious in baking and can be used in biscuits, cream fillings, shortbread and biscotti. Try them too dipped in egg whites and sprinkled with salt, cinnamon and a little sugar and baked in the oven for a Christmas treat. Almond nut butter is delicious as is almond and chia seed pudding. Fantastic in salads, almonds are amazing mixed with oats and dried fruits to make high energy bars.

Brazil Nuts

Brazil nuts come from a tree that is grown in many parts of the Amazon. They are actually the seeds and the tree grows up to 50m tall. Each tree can provide up to 250lbs of nuts each year. **It is actually illegal in Brazil to cut down a Brazil nut tree as each can live between 500 and 800 years!** Their shells are famously difficult to crack but it is definitely worth it for the nut inside is deliciously tender and rich. Brazil nuts are high in heart healthy fats and protein, antioxidants, fibre, vitamins and minerals.

However, it is the high selenium content of Brazil nuts that sets them aside from all others. Selenium is often hard to get from our everyday diets but not anymore. Brazil nuts are the number one food source on the planet for selenium with just two nuts per day being sufficient and far more effective than any supplement. Selenium contains

Cinnamon, Vanilla and Brazil Nut Vegan Butter

Ingredients

3 cups of raw Brazil nuts

The seeds from 1 vanilla bean pod

2 tablespoons maple syrup

1 tablespoon ground cinnamon

1 teaspoon salt

Preheat the oven to 170°C and place the Brazil nuts onto a lined baking tray and roast in the oven for 12 minutes, turning half way through – be careful they do not burn. Remove and allow to cool.

Place the nuts with all remaining ingredients into a food processor or blender and blend until smooth and creamy – you may need to scrape down the sides of the blender several times during this process but believe me it is worth it.

anti-inflammatory properties and defends against free radical damage. It has also been scientifically proven to lift moods and prevent depression. As the thyroid gland has more selenium per gram of tissue than any other organ of the body, regular consumption of Brazil nuts may help to regulate thyroid function and protect the thyroid.

Like many nuts, Brazil nuts are rich in ellagic acid which is highly anti-inflammatory and their combination of potassium, calcium, magnesium and of course selenium helps to maintain a healthy blood pressure. This coupled with their healthy fats which aids healthy cholesterol levels, makes them a real heart health booster.

Uses – Apart from eating them raw or blanched, they can be roasted, shaved and crushed to add to other foods. Brazil nut butter is deliciously rich and Brazil nut milk is a great alternative to regular or soy milk. Brazil nut roast is always popular and not just with the vegetarians. Brazil nuts work fabulously with cookies and sweet treats, and can be used to make a Brazil nut pesto. Cauliflower, carrot and Brazil nut soup is divine.

Take note – It is possible to overdose on Brazil nuts, leading to selenium toxicity. Symptoms include diarrhoea, coughing, hair loss, nausea, brittle nails. Therefore, it is best to stick to the recommended daily serving of one to six nuts.

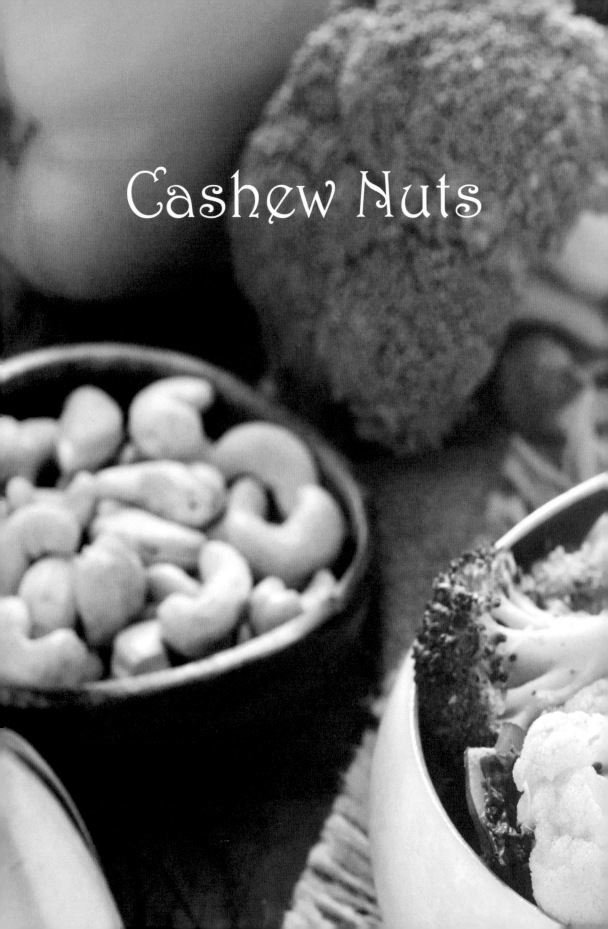

Cashew Nuts

Cashew, Coconut and Date Bars

Ingredients

¼ cup of raw almonds
½ cup of shaved coconut
10 pitted dates

¼ cup of cashew nuts
1 teaspoon of coconut oil

Blend the almonds and coconut in a food processor then add the dates and pulse until combined.

Add the cashew nuts and coconut oil and once again pulse until you have a thick, sticky mixture. Line a square tin with greaseproof paper and pour the mixture into the tin.

Cover with another layer of greaseproof paper and press down to flatten and make smooth.

Chill for a minimum of 30 minutes then slice into bars.

Cashew nuts are the third most consumed tree nut in the world. Native to Brazil, they are now cultivated in more than 30 countries. Rich in antioxidants and cholesterol free, they have a much lower fat content than most other nuts and the fat they contain is oleic acid (the super healthy one found in olive oil). They also contain high levels of iron, magnesium, selenium, phosphorous and zinc; their health benefits are numerous. Studies have shown they may reduce the risk of cancer, and they also aid the reduction of blood pressure, muscle soreness and fatigue. They support the nervous system, are good for the heart and boost bone strength.

Uses – Always popular in curries and Indian dishes, I love to add cashews to stir fries or to roast them with broccoli or other vegetables. They make a fantastic crust for beef, and work well with noodles and rice dishes or as a crumble topping for fruit. And I have to say, cashew nut butter is just about the most creamy and delicious treat in the world, and I often end up eating it straight from the jar!

Interesting Fact – Roasting cashew nuts actually increases the level of nutrients compared to eating them raw.

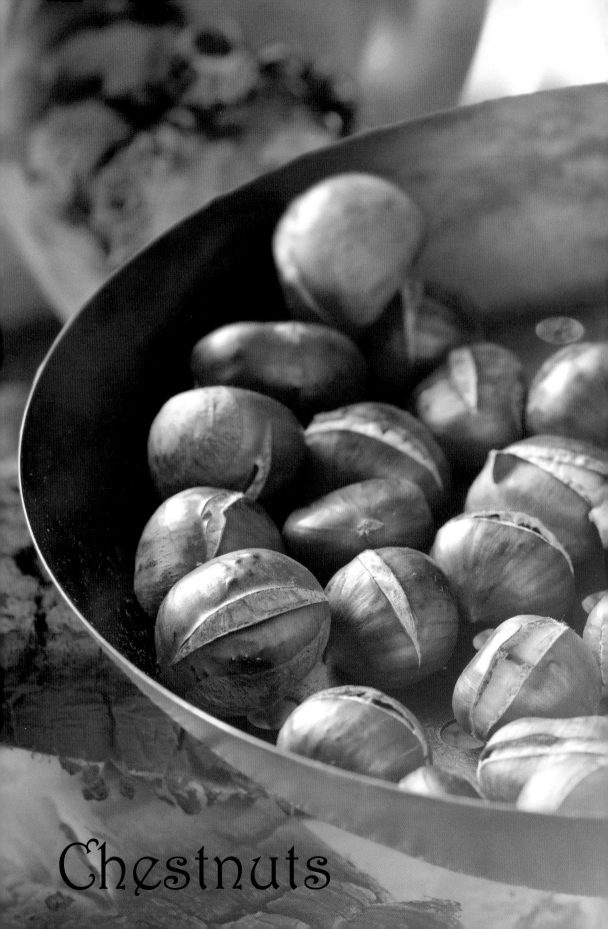

Chestnuts

Chestnut Lentil Stew

Ingredients

4 carrots peeled and diced

3 celery stalks diced

2 onions diced

5 garlic cloves minced

1 litre vegetable stock

1 400g tin chopped tomatoes

1 400g tin lentils drained and
 rinsed

300g cooked peeled chestnuts

Salt and pepper for seasoning

1 tablespoon of mixed dried herbs

1 teaspoon of butter

1 tablespoon oil

1 tablespoon of tomato puree

Heat both the oil and butter in a large saucepan and add the carrots, onion and celery and cook over a medium heat for around 15 to 20 minutes.

Add the tomato puree and cook for a further two to three minutes before adding the minced garlic and cooking for three to four minutes more.

Add the stock and tomatoes, stir well then simmer for 30 minutes.

Add the herbs, chestnuts, lentils with a little salt and pepper then cook for one hour until the chestnuts are soft.

Well given that Christmas just happens to be my favourite time of the year, simply hearing the word chestnuts makes me smile and think of that wonderful Frank Sinatra song. But don't save them just for the festive season as these nuts have an awful lot to offer and deserve their place in my list of super nuts. They contain far less fat than most nuts, yet they are still very nutritious. Chestnuts are actually an excellent source of vitamin C with just 100g of nuts containing almost three-quarters of our daily recommended intake which helps to boost the immune system, aid the formation of collagen and protect from harmful free radicals. They are a super source of Vitamin B too. They are also rich in fibre and folates as well as those heart healthy monounsaturated acids which lower cholesterol and reduce the risk of heart disease and stroke. Chestnuts include an excellent combination of the minerals iron, magnesium, manganese, potassium and zinc which together help to lower blood pressure, boost the immune system, promote healthy bones, aid muscle and joint recovery and reduce the risk of migraines.

Uses – Obviously you have to roast them on an open fire at Christmas but their sweet, earthy flavour means they work well in a range of dishes, from soups, salads, stews, stuffing, risotto, cakes, and pasta pesto. I love serving them with Brussels sprouts and bacon.

Hazelnuts

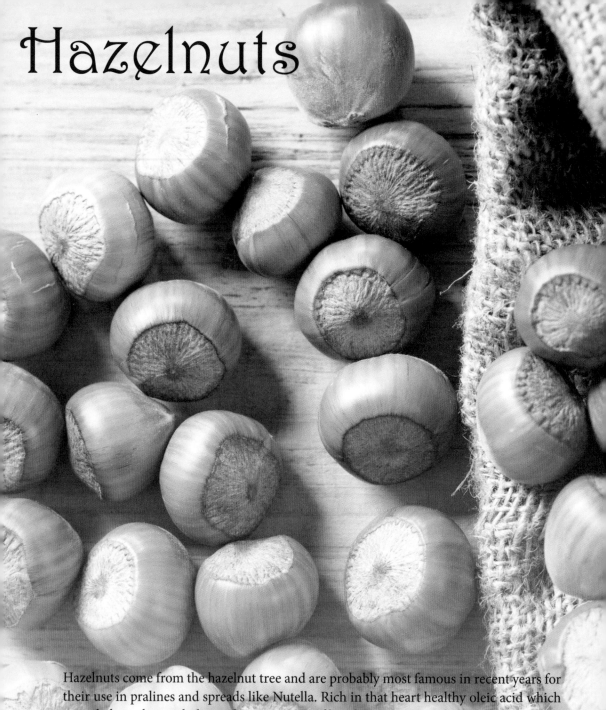

Hazelnuts come from the hazelnut tree and are probably most famous in recent years for their use in pralines and spreads like Nutella. Rich in that heart healthy oleic acid which again helps to lower cholesterol, just one cup of hazelnuts also provides almost half of our recommended daily intake of magnesium. They are also an excellent source of vitamin E, which promotes healthy skin and prevents ageing as well as vitamin B6 which supports the nervous system and brain.

Studies have shown that hazelnuts are one of the highest natural sources of antioxidants. They are high in fibre, supporting the digestive system and preventing constipation. Hazelnuts have also been shown be effective in preventing urinary tract infections (due to their proanthocyanidin content), diabetes and kidney stones as well as controlling blood

Hazelnut Beef Stir Fry

Ingredients

1lb of beef cut into thin strips
2 tablespoons of oil
2 teaspoons of corn flour
2 tablespoons of Teriyaki sauce
1 green pepper sliced

2 carrots sliced
6 spring onions sliced
¾ cup or roasted chopped
  hazelnuts

Mix the Teriyaki sauce, corn flour and one tablespoon of oil and add the beef strips. Leave to marinate for 30 minutes.

Heat the remaining tablespoon of oil in a hot pan, remove the beef from the marinade but keep the sauce.

Add the beef to the pan with the vegetables and cook until the meat is browned and the vegetables are tender.

Add the marinade to the pan and continue cooking until the sauce has thickened.

Next put the hazelnuts in the pan and stir then serve with rice or green vegetables.

pressure and also preventing depression. Just one handful of hazelnuts provides one third of your daily iron requirement as well as minerals including magnesium, calcium and potassium.

Uses – Hazelnuts make a delicious spread when blended and then mixed with cacao, and they are wonderful used as a stuffing for mushrooms, and hazelnut vinaigrette is most popular. Try using them in dumplings, experiment with hazelnut and pumpkin bread or beef and hazelnut stir fry. Or add them to homemade coleslaws or even lettuce leaf wraps. Hazelnut blue cheese dressing has to be sampled and hazelnut caramel brownies are simply special.

Interesting Fact – Studies have shown that hazelnuts are actually one of the highest natural sources of antioxidants.

Macadamias

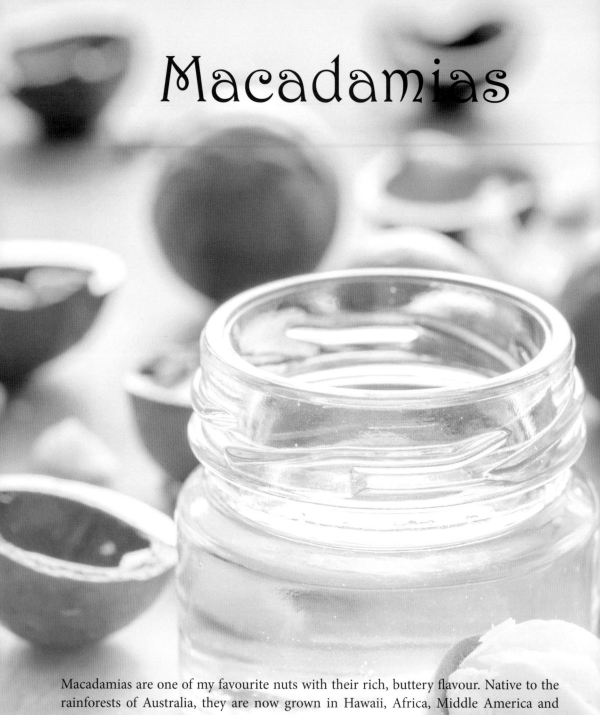

Macadamias are one of my favourite nuts with their rich, buttery flavour. Native to the rainforests of Australia, they are now grown in Hawaii, Africa, Middle America and Brazil. Macadamias have the highest fat, lowest protein and carbohydrate content of all the nuts. However, their fat is the monounsaturated fat which is the heart healthy fat and may be beneficial if you want to lower cholesterol levels. They are an excellent source of fibre too with just 100g providing almost one quarter of your daily recommended intake, and they also contain high levels of calcium, selenium, magnesium, iron and zinc. Rich in B vitamins, they are also a good source of vitamins A and E, which are excellent antioxidants and protect our cells from free radicals.

Macadamia Crusted Fish

Ingredients

2 eggs
1/8 teaspoon cayenne pepper
1 cup all-purpose flour

1¾ cup of chopped macadamias
1 tablespoon melted butter
4 white fish fillets of choice

Place the eggs and cayenne in a bowl and whisk.

Put the flour in another bowl and the macadamia in a separate bowl.

Take each fish fillet, coat in the flour, then dip in the egg and finally roll in the nuts.

Place each fillet on a lined baking tray, drizzle with the butter then bake at 180°C for around 15 to 20 minutes.

This dish is perfect served with wilted greens and a wedge of lemon.

Uses – Apart from being eaten raw, macadamia nuts make a delicious nut butter which you would struggle not to eat straight from the jar. They also work well in sweet baking such as in cookies, sprinkled over frozen yoghurt or ice cream, and in brownies and macaroons. But don't stop at the sweet stuff – they make a delicious crunchy topping for salmon or try mixing chopped macadamias with shredded coconut, breadcrumbs, paprika and Cajun seasoning. All you need to do is simply dip some jumbo prawns in flour, then in fluffy egg whites and finally in the crunchy, nutty mixture and fry until golden brown – which should take approximately two minutes on each side – then devour.

Interesting Facts – Macadamia trees grow to about 15 metres in height but it takes seven years after plantation before they mature and start to produce fruit. Also, macadamia nuts are toxic to dogs!

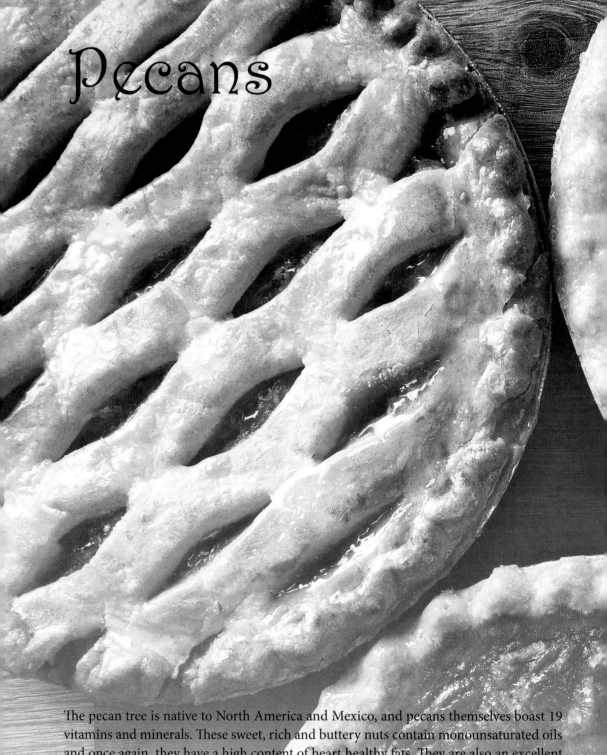

Pecans

The pecan tree is native to North America and Mexico, and pecans themselves boast 19 vitamins and minerals. These sweet, rich and buttery nuts contain monounsaturated oils and once again, they have a high content of heart healthy fats. They are also an excellent source of fibre, boosting digestive and colon health and preventing constipation. Pecans contain oleic acid which has been shown to reduce the risk of breast cancer. They are also rich in phosphorous which apart from clearing waste from the body and aiding recovery post-exercise, is vital for the growth and repair of cells and tissues and promotes healthy bones and teeth.

Pecan Rice

Ingredients

1 cup of brown rice
2 tablespoons butter
¼ cup of onion finely chopped
½ cup of chopped pecans
2 tablespoons of parsley minced

¼ teaspoon of dried ginger
¼ teaspoon dried basil
¼ teaspoon salt
¼ teaspoon of black pepper

Bring two cups of water to the boil, add the rice, stir and cover and leave to cook for around 40 minutes until all the water is absorbed and the rice is cooked.

Towards the end of the cooking of the rice, melt the butter in a pan and add all remaining ingredients.

Cook over a medium heat for four to five minutes until the onions are soft. Stir this mixture into the rice and serve.

They contain high levels of magnesium too, helping to relax muscles and providing anti-inflammatory effects. Studies have shown that by consuming just 100mg of magnesium each day reduces the risk of stroke by nine per cent and it has also been linked to lowering blood pressure. Pecans are rich in phytochemicals, or natural compounds, which protect the body from damaging free radicals and diseases. They are also a good source of manganese, a fantastic immune booster that may aid brain health. Bursting with anti-ageing antioxidants, they help to keep wrinkles away and also contain a super source of L Arginine which is an amino acid that has been shown to treat baldness and stimulate hair growth.

Uses – Pecans work fantastically with both sweet and savoury dishes. I am sure you will all know of the famous pecan pie, but these wonderful nuts can also be add to salads, sprinkled over mashed sweet potatoes and dabbed with butter and baked until crispy. They are perfect for making a banana loaf, make great toppings for muffins, and are delicious, and I love them in homemade oat bars or granolas.

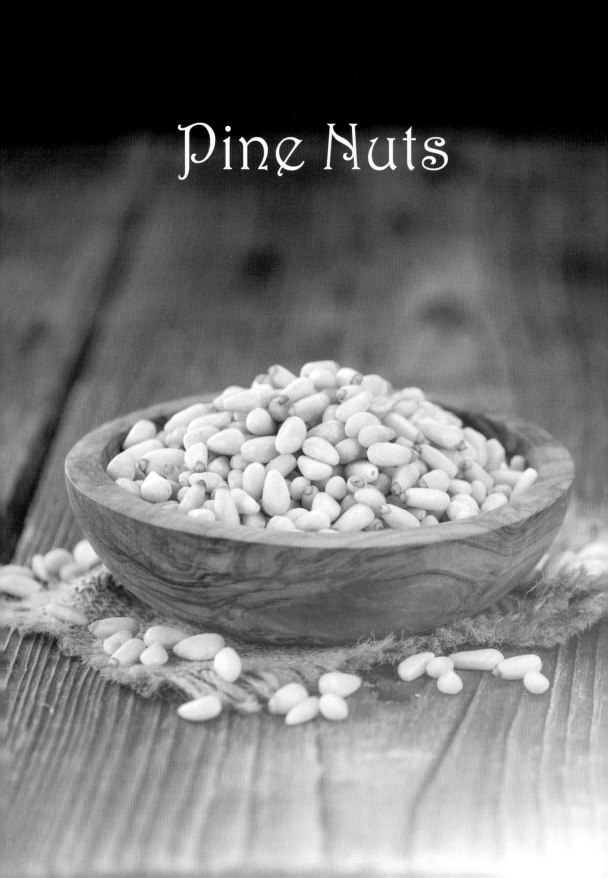

Pine Nuts

Broccoli and Asparagus Salad

Ingredients

12 spears of thick asparagus
1 large handful of broccoli florets
2 tablespoons lemon juice
1 shallot chopped finely
3 tablespoons of extra virgin olive
   oil

¼ cup of pine nuts toasted
A handful of radishes finely sliced
The zest of one lemon
Parmesan for garnishing

Whisk together the lemon juice, salt, shallots and olive oil. Add the pine nuts, mix and set aside.

Heat a little oil in a pan over a high heat and add the asparagus and broccoli and cook for a couple of minutes until they are slightly charred but still have 'bite'.

Remove from the heat and stir in the radish and lemon zest.

Toss with the dressing and plate up. Sprinkle with parmesan.

Most people do not realize that pine nuts are actually the small seeds of the pine cone and are found most commonly in India, Afghanistan and Pakistan. They are another excellent source of monounsaturated fats which help to lower bad cholesterol and raise good cholesterol. With their high levels of protein, they provide instant and slow burning energy and also aid the repair and building of muscles. Rich in antioxidants, they protect the body from damaging free radicals, illness and diseases as well as slowing down the ageing process. They contain beta carotene and lutein which are good for eye health and their rich vitamin E content also promotes healthy skin.

Uses – Their fabulous sweet buttery flavour of pine nuts makes them a wonderful addition to so many recipes. Popular in pesto, casseroles, curries, or added to pasta, salads, yoghurt, ice cream, cookies and granola, we always top our homemade soups with toasted pine nuts which by the way makes the kitchen smell amazing!

Pistachios

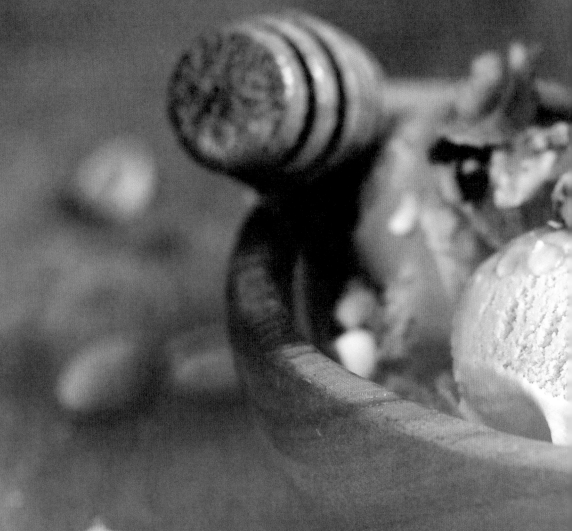

I adore pistachios and there has been many a day in our house where a rather large pile of empty shells has resulted from a pistachio nut snack attack! Pistachios are actually the kernels that come from the fruit of the Pistacia plant which is a broad bushy tree native to West Asia and Turkey. After plantation it actually takes between eight and ten years for the plant to produce its first crop. Pistachios are a rich source of antioxidant phytochemicals such as carotene and vitamin E, so they help to fight the damage done to the body from free radicals and protecting it from diseases and infections.

Super rich in B vitamins, their high level of monounsaturated fatty acids may aid the lowering of cholesterol and thus reduce the risk of coronary heart disease and stroke. They are an excellent source of protein and energy, and a recent study showed that

Pistachio Crusted Scallops

Ingredients

2 tablespoons unsalted butter

2 tablespoons or raw shelled pistachios

1 tablespoon of chopped fresh thyme

1 tablespoon of chopped fresh tarragon

1 tablespoon of chopped fresh chives

8 large sea scallops with the side muscle removed

Salt and pepper to season and oil for cooking

Melt one tablespoon of butter in a pan over a medium heat and add the pistachios. Cook for two to three minutes. Then remove from the heat and allow the mixture to cool.

Once cooled, completely chop the nuts and toss in a bowl with the chives, tarragon and thyme.

Season the scallops with salt and pepper, heat the remaining tablespoon of butter in the pan and add the scallops.

Cook for around two minutes of each side until they are golden brown on the outside.

diets containing pistachios actually reduced blood pressure in a trial of adults with high cholesterol. And just to prove that healthy fats are good for you, and definitely not something to be avoided, a study in India showed that people who ate pistachios daily for 24 weeks lost 0.7 inches from their waists, reduced their cholesterol, improved blood sugar levels and lowered inflammation.

Uses – Pistachios taste great in cookies, pates, granolas, salads, pasta dishes and as a crunchy topping for chicken. And of course, let's not forget pistachio ice cream!

Interesting Fact – In ancient times, pistachios were the symbol of wellbeing and robust health.

Walnuts

Walnuts have been part of the human diet for thousands of years and since ancient times they have been seen as the symbol of intelligence with their resemblance to the human brain. Their high Omega-3 content makes them a heart healthy warrior, helping to lower cholesterol and blood pressure. Omega-3 fatty acids have also been linked to a reduced risk of coronary heart disease as well as strokes. **Just a quarter of a cup of walnuts provides us with more than 100 per cent of our recommended daily intake of Omega-3 fats and huge amounts of copper, manganese, biotin and molybdenum.**

Their high antioxidant content helps to fight inflammation, ageing and many diseases and illnesses, and walnuts are also a skin super food, just bursting with vitamin E. They also contain high levels of L Arginine and so boost hair health, and they are also rich in B vitamins, manganese, calcium, iron, potassium and zinc. They really are an all-round energy and health boosting snack.

Walnut Honey Mustard Chicken Strips

Ingredients

1lb boneless chicken breast fillets
¼ cup yellow mustard
¼ cup of honey
1 cup of breadcrumbs
¼ cup of walnuts
2 tablespoons fresh parsley

½ teaspoon salt
¼ teaspoon pepper
To make the dipping sauce:
¼ cup of yellow mustard
¼ cup of honey

Preheat the oven to 180°C. Mix together the honey and mustard and set aside.

Place the breadcrumbs, walnuts, parsley, salt and pepper into a food processor and blend until they form fine bread crumbs. Place in a bowl.

Put a wire cooling rack on top of a baking tray and brush or spray with oil. Taking each strip of chicken at a time, dip into the honey and mustard mixture then roll in the breadcrumb mixture before sitting onto the cooling rack. Repeat until all chicken strips are coated and placed on the rack.

Place in the oven and cook for 20 minutes. Remove from the oven and change the setting to grill. Grill the strips for three minutes on each side until golden and crispy.

Mix the honey and mustard for the dip together until fully combined then serve in pots with the chicken strips.

Uses – Walnut butter is very popular as are walnuts in breads, general baking, salads, granolas and pies. Walnuts work wonderfully with rice dishes, roasted or stir fried vegetables, frittatas and especially with cheeses. I make a pasta dish with blue cheese and walnuts, and there are no words good enough to describe it!

Interesting Fact – The white flaky, almost waxy outer part of the shelled walnut, is a little bitter but it is thought to contain up to 90 per cent of the nutrients – so no peeling!

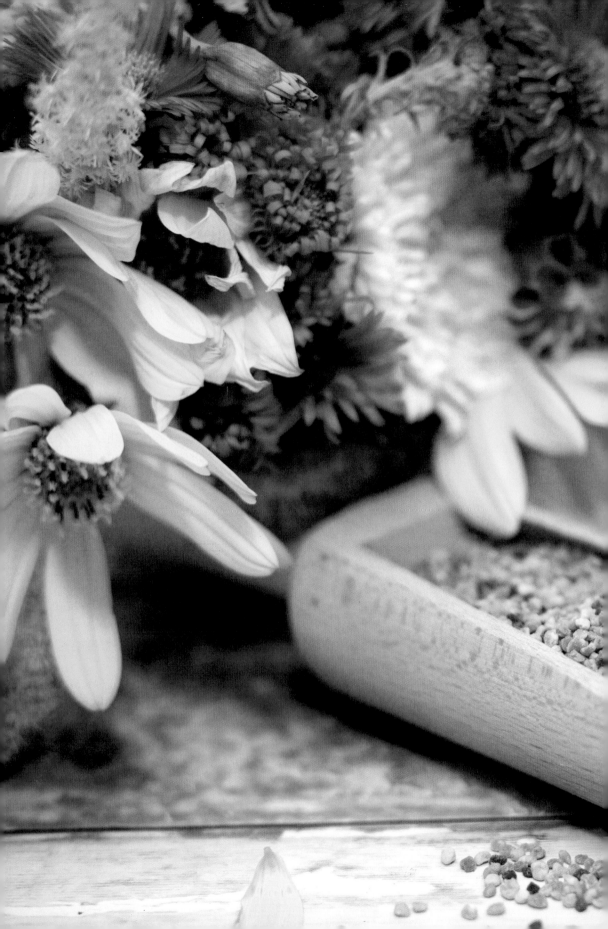

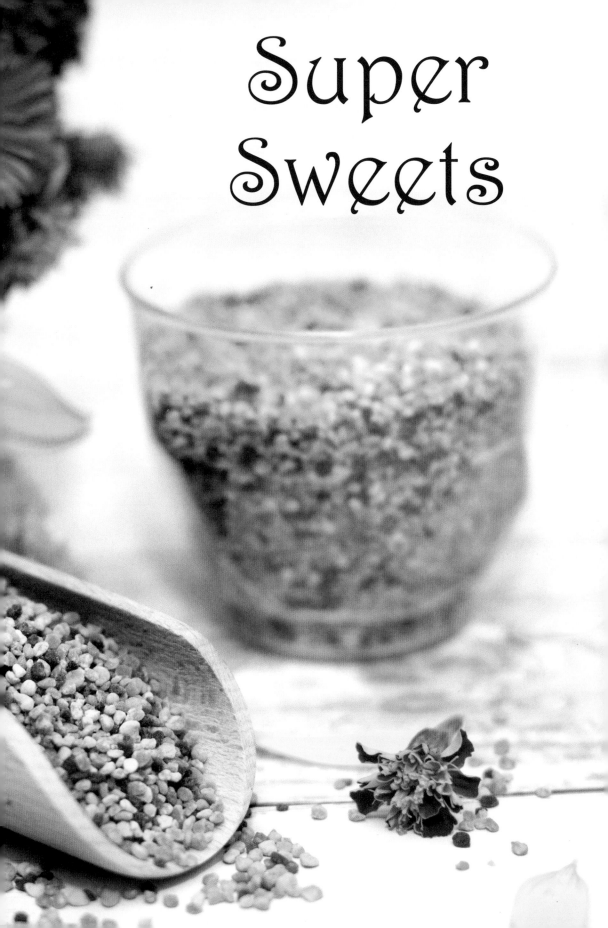

Super Sweets

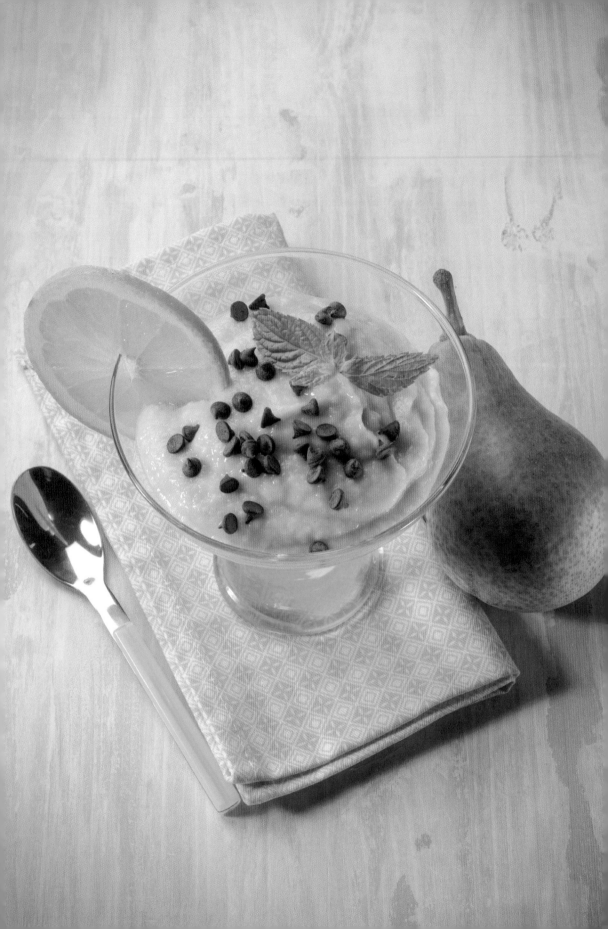

No, I am afraid this section is not about to prove that Haribos really are superfoods. However, it will demonstrate that there are some fabulous sweet and healthy foods out there that really do taste too good to be true. Desserts do not have to be naughty, and nutritious certainly does not have to mean bland. Adding my super sweet foods into your diet will not only tantalize your taste buds, it will benefit your body and mind too.

I think before we continue with this section, it is worth stressing why refined sugar really should be avoided and replaced with my super sweets.

According to the World Health Organisation, sugar should only equate to five per cent of our daily calorie consumption, which is only around 25g for an adult of normal weight. That is not very much at all when you consider that one can of cola contains 35g and would put you one third over your daily limit.

To make it clear:

- **Sugar contains no nutrients**
- **Sugar contains no protein**
- **Sugar contains no healthy fats**
- **Sugar contains no enzymes**
- **Sugar contains empty calories, and deprives the body of minerals.**
  Much has been written in the press recently about sugar – but let's examine here what it really does to our bodies.
- **Sugar causes blood glucose to rise and plummet**
  Unstable blood sugar levels cause mood swings, fatigue, headaches and cravings for more sugar. Cravings set the stage for a cycle of addiction in which every new hit of sugar makes you feel better for a few hours, but subsequently results in more cravings and increased hunger.
- **Sugar increases the risk of obesity, diabetes and heart disease**
  Several large studies have shown that the more sugar a person consumes, the greater is their risk of diabetes, heart disease and obesity. New research is also showing a link between sugar and cancer too.
- **Sugar interferes with immune function**
  Bacteria and yeast feed on sugar and when these organisms get out of balance in the body, infections and illnesses are more likely.
- **A high sugar diet often results in chromium deficiency**
  It is a catch 22 situation, if you consume too much sugar and other refined carbohydrates then you will not be getting enough of the trace mineral chromium which regulates blood sugar.
- **Sugar accelerates ageing**
  After hitting the blood stream, sugar attaches itself to proteins in a process called glycation. These new molecular structures contribute to the loss of elasticity found in ageing body tissues, from you skin to your arteries and organs. The more sugar in your blood – the faster the damage takes hold.
- **Sugar causes tooth decay**
  With all the other life threatening effects of sugar, we sometimes forget the most basic damage that it does. Sugar sits on your teeth and creates decay more efficiently than any other substance.
- **Sugar can cause gum disease which has been linked to heart disease**
  Evidence has shown that chronic infections that result from periodontal problems play a role in the development of coronary artery disease.
- **Sugar affects behaviour and cognition in children**
  Between 1979 and 1983, 803 New York City public schools reduced the amount of sugars and artificial sweeteners from the school breakfasts and lunches. A 15.7 per cent increase in academic ranking was the result with no other changes!

- **Sugar increases Stress**

  When we are under stress, our body releases stress hormones to prepare the body for an attack. The exact same thing happens when blood sugar drops. When you eat sugar you have an immediate blood sugar spike which is shorty followed by a dive. This triggers the stress hormone reaction, causing anxiety, irritability and even shakiness.

- **Sugar takes the place of important nutrients**

  Studies show that people who consume the most sugar have the lowest intakes of essential nutrients especially vitamins A, C, B12, calcium, magnesium and iron.

So now you know the harmful effects that sugar has on the body, it is important that you know where it lurks. Food doesn't need to taste sweet to be loaded with sugar. In fact, many processed, packaged and convenience foods are high in sugar and just because a food claims to be 'low fat' or 'diet' or 'low carbs' does not mean it is not high in sugar.

So what should you be looking out for when trying to avoid sugar?

Believe it or not there are 257 different names for forms of sugar – yes really! However, some of the more common ones used on food labels are as follows:

- barley malt
- beet sugar
- brown sugar
- buttered syrup
- cane-juice crystals
- cane sugar
- caramel
- carob syrup
- corn syrup
- corn syrup solids
- dextran
- dextrose
- diatase
- diastatic malt
- ethyl maltol
- fructose
- fruit juice
- fruit juice concentrate
- glucose
- glucose solids
- golden sugar
- golden syrup
- grape sugar
- high-fructose corn syrup
- honey
- invert sugar
- lactose
- malt syrup
- maltodextrin
- maltose
- mannitol
- raw sugar
- refiner's syrup
- sorbitol
- sorghum syrup
- sucrose
- sugar
- turbinado sugar
- yellow sugar

So does that mean that fruit is bad as it can be high in sugar?

Given that I have included a Super Fruits section in this book you probably already know the answer, but just to clarify that fruit is a highly nutritious food. Whilst it does contain natural sugars, it also contains fibre, antioxidants and many nutrients, and fruit is not disproportionately high in sugar by weight compared to say sweets or chocolate.

So now that we have talked about the sugars you should be avoiding, let's concentrate on some healthier, sweet foods.

Bee
Pollen

Bee pollen is the pollen of the young bee and its protein content stands at 40 per cent. In fact, it is richer in protein than any animal source. It is thought to be one of nature's most complete foods containing almost all the nutrients required by humans. Bee pollen is rich in antioxidants which as we now know, help to fight off the damage caused by free radicals. They also reduce inflammation in the body, and boost the immune system. Bee pollen is high in rutin which is a specific bioflavonoid that strengthens blood vessels, and can regulate cholesterol levels and support circulation. Pollen reduces the presence of

Raw Bee Pollen Brownies

Ingredients

1 tablespoon bee pollen

1 cup cacao nibs

1 teaspoon cacao

2 cups of walnuts

1 cup of raw almonds

2½ cups of dates

Pinch of sea salt

Grind the cacao nibs to a fine powder. Roughly chop the dates and almonds. Place the walnuts in a food processor and blend to a fine powder.

Add the bee pollen, salt and cacao powder and combine.

Slowly add the dates until you achieve a crumbly consistency.

Pour into a bowl and add the almonds. Tip this mixture into a baking tin lined with greaseproof and press down. Sprinkle cacao nibs onto the top and press into the mixture.

Place in the freezer for 30 minutes then remove and dust with cacao powder and bee pollen then cut into squares.

histamine and can prevent allergies and allergic reactions. It boosts the hormones been used to help with infertility; and it supports a healthy digestive system and is a fantastic natural energy booster, preventing fatigue.

Uses – I always add a couple of tablespoons of bee pollen granules to my breakfast and it is a great topping on fruit, cereal or homemade granola, and it tastes delicious in smoothies. It is best not to heat it as this diminishes its nutritional benefit, and it is more effective if eaten at mealtimes.

Interesting Fact – Next time you are about to curse a bee think twice as it takes a bee working eight hours a day more than one month to produce one teaspoon of pollen.

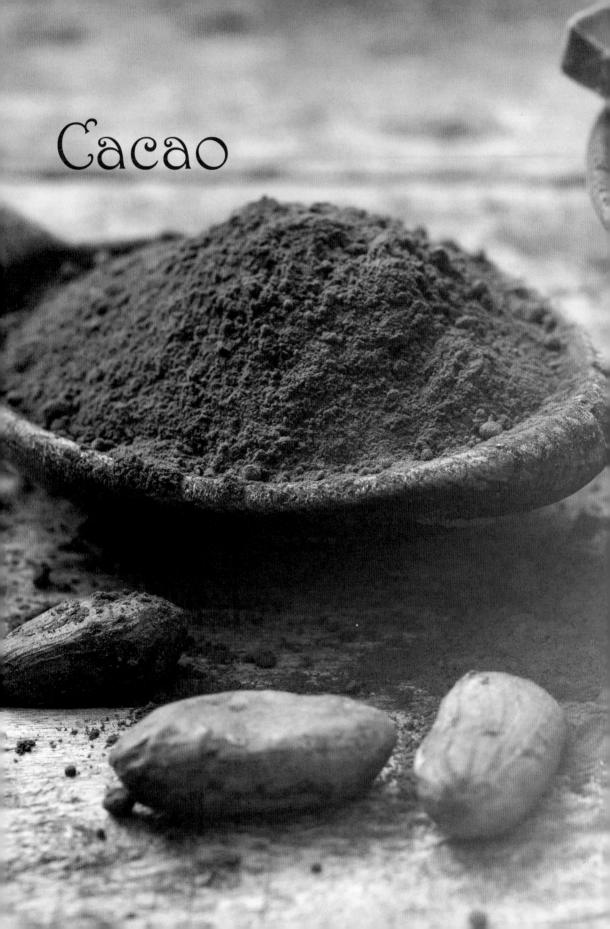

Cacao

Raw Avocado Cacao Mousse

Believe me you really cannot taste the avocado in this, and this dish is so healthy and delicious that you don't even need to save it for dessert – you can have it for breakfast too.

Ingredients

¾ cup almond milk

3 avocados peeled and with the stone removed

1¼ cups of raw cacao powder

¼ cup of agave syrup

Place all the ingredients and blend until smooth. Pour or pipe into glasses and chill overnight. Can be served with fruit or chopped nuts or alone.

Cacoa has so many health benefits that I'm not even sure where to start, but here is the basic low down:

• It is has more iron than any other plant-based food.
• It contains 40 times more antioxidants than blueberries.
• Raw cacoa has more calcium than cow's milk.
• It is rich is magnesium.
• As a mood-booster, it is a natural anti-depressant.

Raw cacoa is rich in protein, carotene, magnesium, thiamine, riboflavin and essential fatty acids. It may help to lower cholesterol, reduce the risk of cancer, boost brain function, and to raise mood and energy levels. Recent studies have revealed that cocoa contains a higher level of antioxidant activity than tea or red wine.

Uses – Now this is the fun part! I love to mix raw cacao powder with coconut oil to make a delicious chocolate spread. Raw avocado and cacao mousse probably doesn't sound that appetizing but it really is AMAZING. Add it to shakes (always popular with children) or have a try at making your own raw chocolate truffles, raw protein balls and healthy caramel pecan pie. Chocolate chia pudding is a delicious and nutritious breakfast and you can use it to add a chocolately twist to granola bars. In fact, any recipe that contains cocoa powder you can simply substitute for raw cacao powder.

Interesting Fact – Cacao and cocoa are not the same thing. Cacao is the tree which produces pods containing beans, and these are used to produce cocoa. But it is the raw cacao which has all the super powers containing four times more antioxidants than regular dark chocolate.

Date Syrup

This is the thick, sweet liquid derived from dates which has recently been shown to have similar antibacterial properties to manuka honey. Tests showed that when the syrup was mixed with a range of disease causing bacteria, including E.coli, it inhibited their growth. It is commonly used in cooking in the Middle East to flavour everything from main courses to desserts. Dates are the fruits that come from the palm tree that originated on the banks of the Nile. They are rich in vitamins, minerals and nutrients, and because they are so effective at replenishing energy and revitalizing the body, they have traditionally been used to break the Ramadan fast.

Oaty Date Bites

Ingredients

200g pitted dates
125g oats
125ml water

2 tablespoons coconut oil as liquid
2 tablespoons date syrup

Preheat the oven to 180°C

Chop the dates then place in a pan with the 125ml water and bring to the boil and simmer for 15 minutes until you have a thick paste.

Add the oats, oil, syrup and a pinch of salt and stir well. Pour the mixture into a lined baking tin ad press to flatten evenly then bake in the oven for 15 to 20 minutes.

I like to slice it whilst still warm in the pan then leave to cool a little before transferring to a wire rack to cool fully.

There are many other 'super' ways to sweeten your food but they fall into another category so let's move on promptly whilst those taste buds are flowing.

Bursting with fibre and antioxidants, as well as flavonoids, and iron, they are a good source of potassium, and help the body to maintain healthy blood pressure levels. Dates are also rich in calcium, magnesium, manganese and copper, helping to aid the production of red blood cells, boost bone health and relax muscles and blood vessels. They also contain high levels of B vitamins which support a healthy nervous system.

Uses – Try making date syrup caramel sauce or wrap whole dates with bacon and drizzle with the syrup. Date and walnut bars are delicious, the syrup can be added to your porridge or you can experiment with sticky date pudding or use the syrup to glaze chicken and top with sesame seeds.

Manuka Honey

And once again it is time to give thanks to those wonderful little creatures called bees! Honey has been used for centuries for medicinal purposes but manuka honey is not the same as any other raw honey. This honey is special! Produced in New Zealand by bees that pollinate the manuka bush, this special honey contains hydrogen peroxide, compounds that provide extra antibacterial strength. You will often notice on the jars of manuka honey that they are graded according to their UMF which is their unique manuka factor or anti-bacterial potency. Manuka honey is expensive but definitely worth the investment. To maximise its benefits it is worth purchasing +UMF 15 or higher. Manuka honey contains more than four times the nutritional benefit of regular honey. It has been shown to improve digestion and reflux as well as preventing infection and speeding up healing when used on wounds. Many hospitals are now applying manuka honey to dressings after surgery. It is also believed to ease eczema and psoriasis symptoms when applied directly to the affected areas, and can be used to treat burns and ulcers.

If you add mauka honey to milk before bedtime, it will promote restful sleep, and taken daily, it will help to boost vitality and skin tone and to reduce food allergies. This wonder

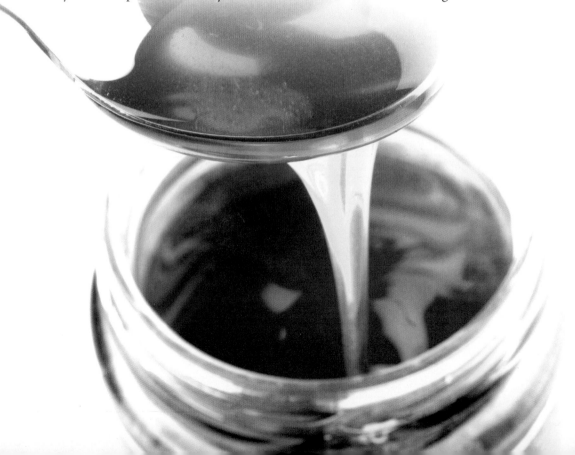

Manuka Honey Granola

Ingredients

150g manuka honey
60ml groundnut oil
250g rolled oats
100g bran
150g sunflower seeds
150g dates chopped

100g hazelnuts roasted and
  chopped
100g apricots chopped
100g wheatgerm
100g sultanas

Preheat the oven to 180°C. Place the oil and honey in a pan and heat on low until the honey has melted.

Add the oats, bran and sunflower seeds to a bowl and mix before pouring on the honey mixture and stirring well.

Spread this mixture onto a baking tray and place in the oven for 25 minutes, stirring every five minutes.

Once it is cooled, place in an airtight container. This will keep for up to a month.

honey has been proven to improve the symptoms of IBS and colitis and is an amazing cough remedy. It can be used to treat dandruff, hair loss, athlete's foot and ringworm. And proving that not all sweet things are bad for our teeth, manuka honey can reduce plaque, promote healthy gums and cut the risk of cavities. Being rich in amino acids, B complex vitamins and minerals such as iron, zinc, magnesium, calcium, copper and potassium it is an all- round immune system and health booster.

Uses – As well as the manuka honey and milk bedtime drink or manuka honey and chamomile tea which is simply wonderful, and my daughter's favourite drink, it can be used in honey barbecue sauce, or honey coleslaw. It is good in cakes, granola, yogurt and fresh fruit too.

Interesting Fact – Archaeologists claim that when they were excavating the tombs of ancient Egyptian royals, they found jars of unspoiled honey in pots.

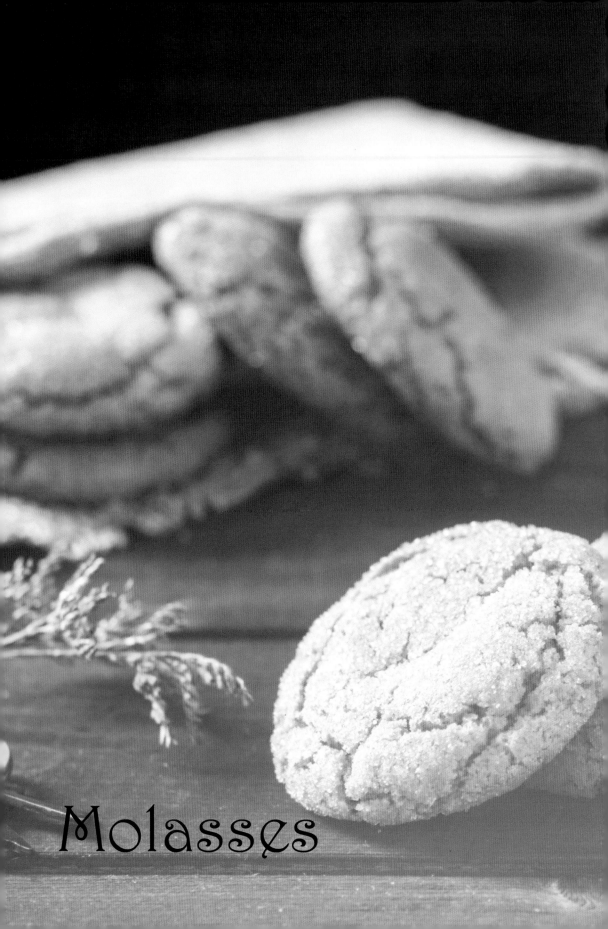

Molasses

Molasses Baked Squash

Ingredients

1 whole squash
2 teaspoons molasses
Pinch cinnamon
Pinch salt

Pinch pepper
I teaspoon butter
2 whole cloves

Heat the oven to 200°C. Wash the squash and cut in half lengthways and remove the seeds.

Mix the remaining ingredients in a bowl and then spread equally over the two halves.

Place onto a baking tray and cover and bake in the oven for 45 minutes. Uncover and bake for a further 10 to 15 minutes until the squash is golden.

Whilst being a sugar cane product, blackstrap molasses contain a wide range of vital vitamins and minerals. It also has the lowest sugar content of all sugar cane products. Molasses is actually the thick, dark syrup that is produced when the sugar cane plant is processed to make refined sugar. It contains all the wonderful vitamins and minerals absorbed by the plant from the soil. Although it still contains a significant amount of sugar which should be kept in mind, it is also an excellent source of iron, manganese, calcium, potassium, magnesium and copper – and is both cholesterol and fat free.

It is often prescribed by doctors to people suffering from anaemia because it has such high iron levels – also important for healthy hair, skin and nails. One to two tablespoons daily mixed in warm water has been proven to help alleviate constipation, and for centuries it has been used to treat PMS. It is a fantastic bone boosting food and its potassium content may help to lower and regulate blood pressure too. It also has an excellent antioxidant profile, and is used to diminish the effects of arthritis. Finally the B vitamins and magnesium it contains promote a healthy nervous system and aid relaxation.

Uses – I'm afraid I cannot advise you to eat your body weight in treacle toffee, but there are some healthy ways to incorporate molasses into your diet. It can be used to make homemade barbecue sauce or baked beans. It is good added to porridge and bananas, or used in fruit cakes, cookies, or good old-fashioned gingerbread but it also makes a fabulous glaze for pork and I love it with roasted carrots and onions.

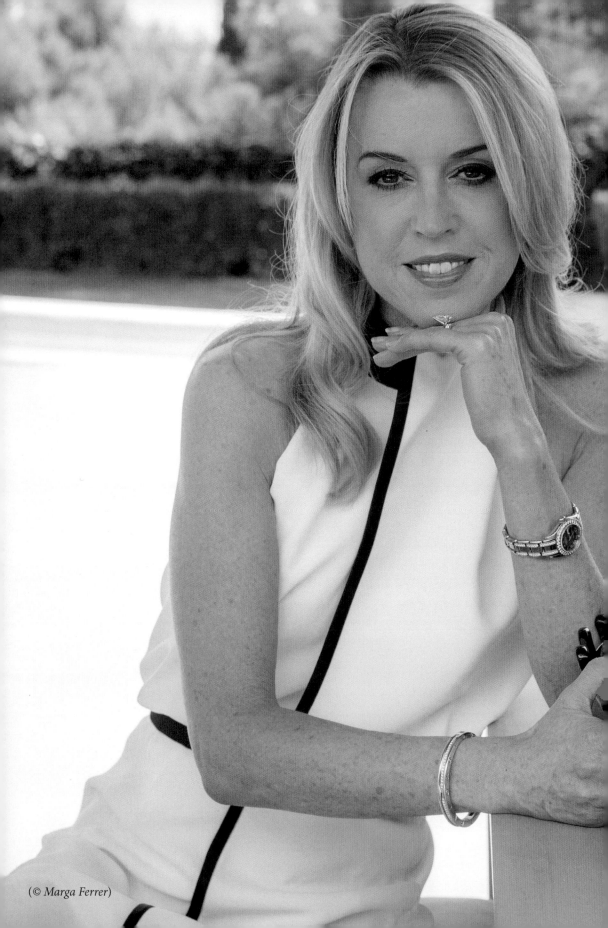

(© Marga Ferrer)

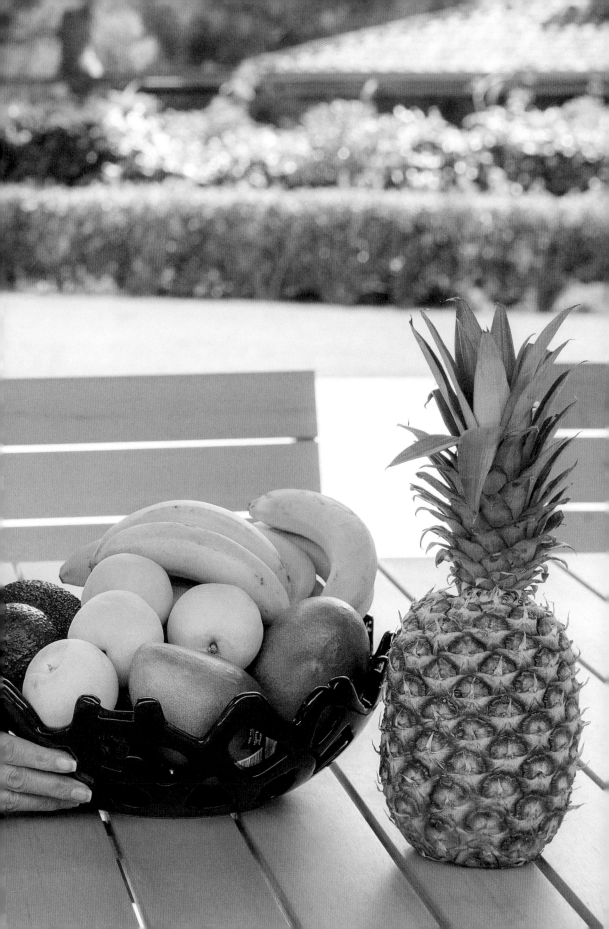

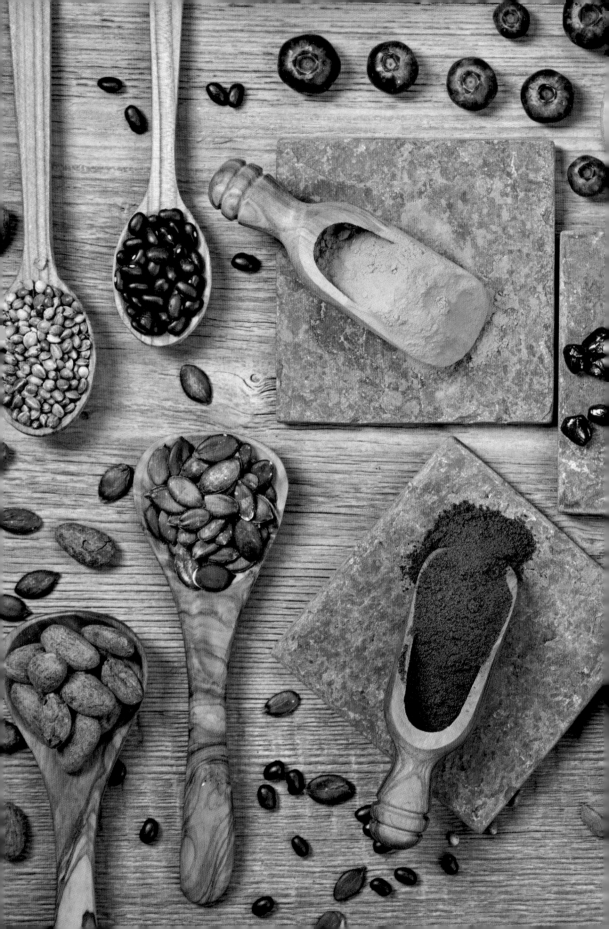

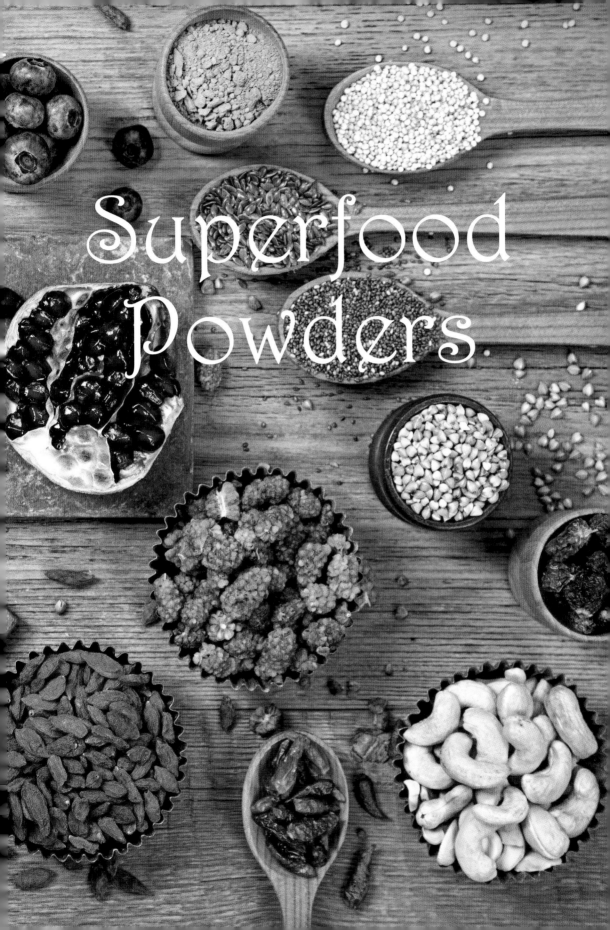

Superfood Powders

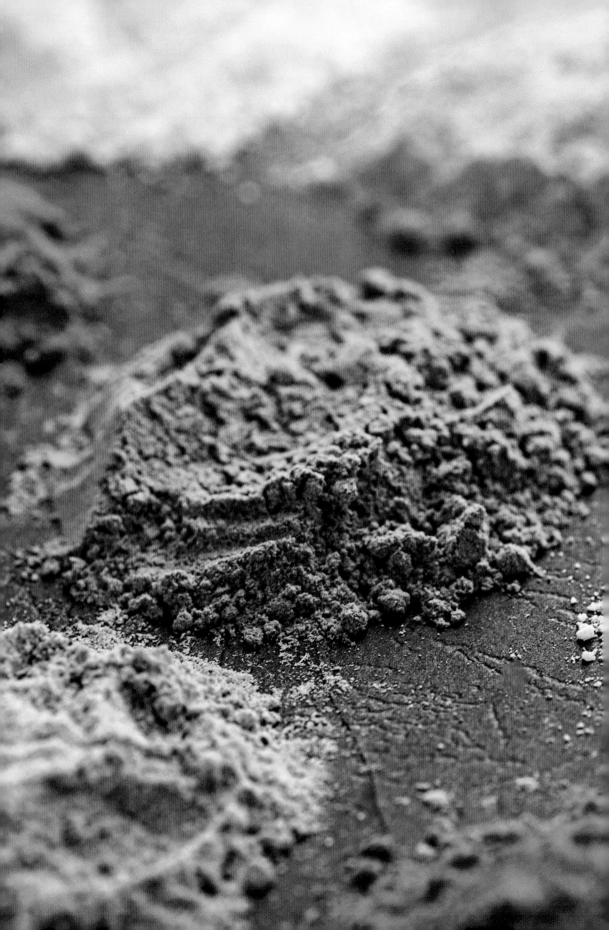

Now this is the section that I have been waiting for and one that I have studied for many years with interest and excitement. I have trialled many of the products listed below and incorporated many of them into my family's diet and I have great faith and belief in these powders.

So from my experience in the health food retail market, I quickly came to realize that often people will read about a new superfood powder in the press, and will go along to their local health food store to buy it, take it home then not know how to use it. Believe me, while it may often be difficult to pronounce the names of some of these powders, or to remember their history or origin, it certainly isn't difficult to add them into your diet. In fact, they not only have numerous health benefits but most definitely add flavour too.

Superfood powders are a dried version of a superfood in its raw, natural state that have been carefully processed or freeze dried to keep all their nutritional qualities intact. They are extremely powerful and potent and are an excellent way to incorporate vitamins, minerals, antioxidants, fibre, protein and micronutrients (the vitamins and minerals we need in small quantities) into our diets.

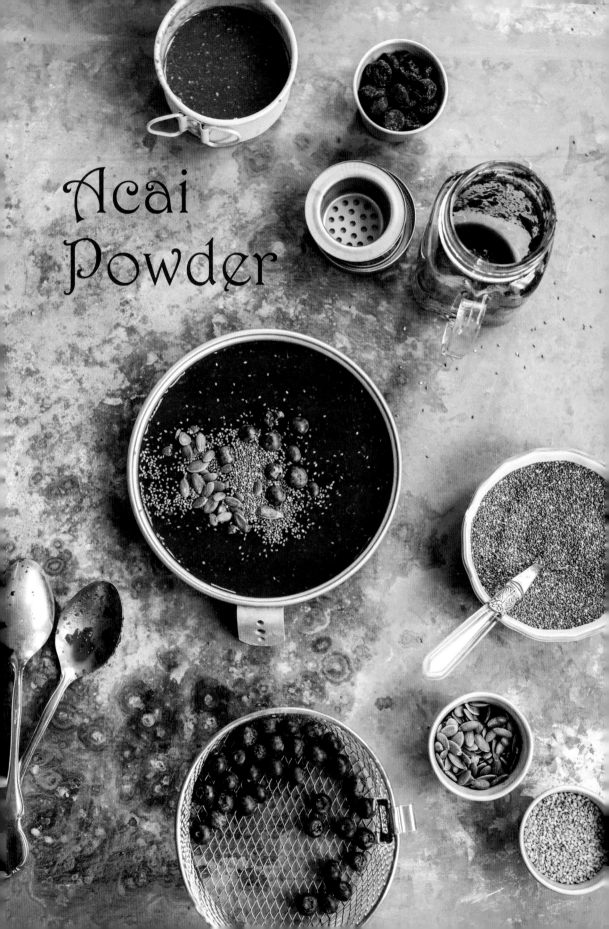

Acai
Powder

Acai are berries that grow on palm trees in Brazil. They are deep purple in colour and similar in size and shape to grapes. The acai berry is best known for its phenomenal antioxidant content. In fact, it is one of the world's highest rated ORAC foods (oxygen radical absorption capacity). ORAC measures just how well the antioxidants neutralize the damaging free radicals in the body. Acai has more than double the antioxidants of blueberries and ten times that of grapes. Anthocyanins are the type of antioxidants found in acai which are particularly beneficial for heart health and may assist in regulating cholesterol levels. These berries are rich in fibre, which helps to promote a healthy digestive system and the removal of waste and toxins from the body, and amino acids which boost energy, strength and performance. The powder is an excellent source of vitamins, calcium, magnesium, zinc and copper and essential fatty acids, making it good for the bones and both the immune and nervous systems.

Uses – Acai is most popular in a range of smoothies but don't stop there, as the powder can be used to make super healthy chocolately muffins or truffles, and a super powered alternative to regular ice cream, fudge or even jam!

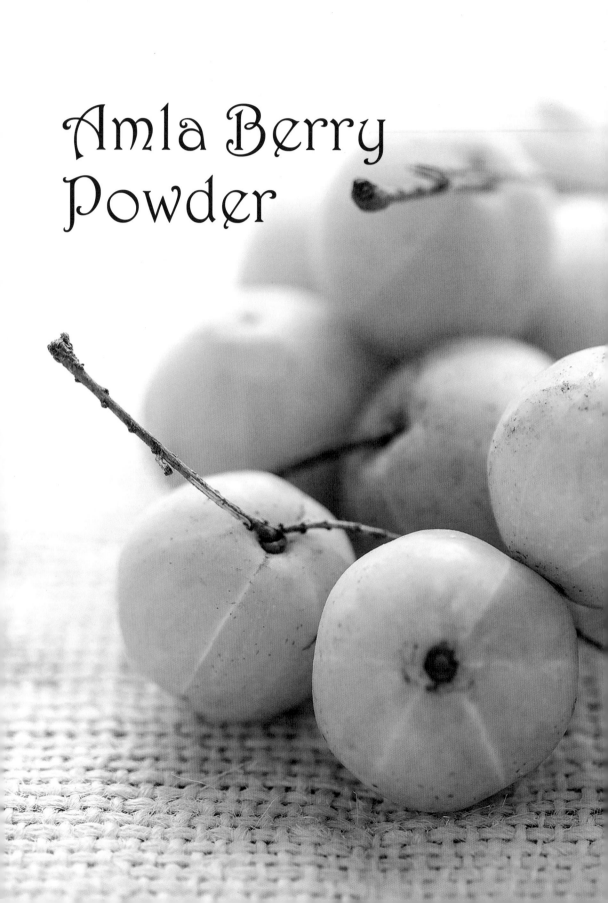

Amla Berry Powder

Amla Berries, otherwise known as Indian gooseberries, ripen in the autumn and are a very nourishing, yet sour fruit. However, they have a very long list of health benefits as they are rich in vitamin C, B vitamins, calcium, phosphorous, iron, carotene and antioxidants. Their high carotene content can help to improve eyesight whilst reducing age-related degeneration. They helps the body to absorb calcium and its protein content aids muscle development, growth and repair. This powder, which works well in pickles, chutneys and Indian dishes, has been shown to be effective in treating PMS as well as effective in treating diabetes due to its high chromium levels. A definite heart healthy ingredient, it is excellent at flushing toxins and waste out of the body, reducing free radicals, and protecting the body from illness. It also helps to promote the growth of healthy hair and prevent hair loss.

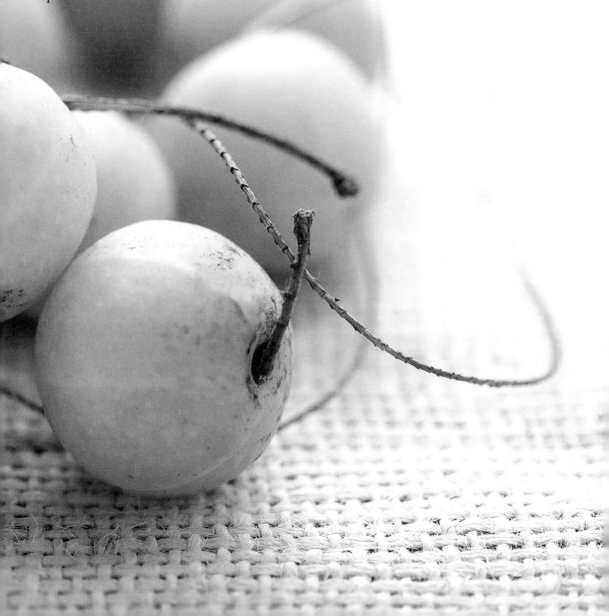

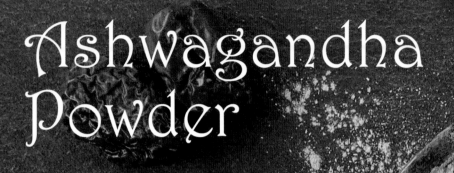
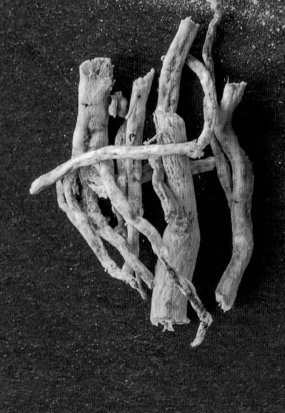

Ashwagandha Powder

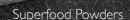

Ashwagandha is an herb, and is often referred to as 'Indian ginseng', and is thought to be an adaptogen – a natural substance that is thought to help the body deal with stress. This herb is often used to boost the immune system, alleviate the symptoms of fatigue, lower cholesterol, aid the digestive system, treat diabetes and also reduce the symptoms of arthritis and other inflammatory diseases. Some studies have suggested that it might be as effective in treating anxiety as medication. It may also reduce depression. Plus it is thought to boost energy, fight infection, and reduce cortisol levels (stress hormones) – less cortisol means less belly fat!!

Uses – Add to warm milk and drink before bed to aid restful sleep or to reduce anxiety. Boil in water for fifteen minutes to make tea. **Note – avoid use if pregnant.**

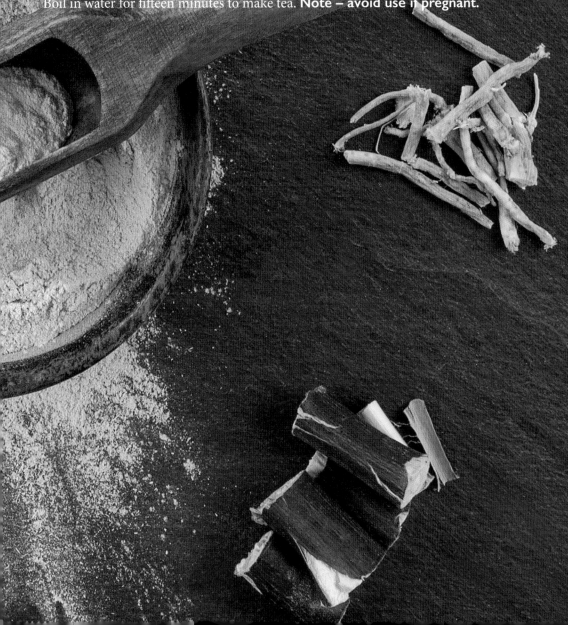

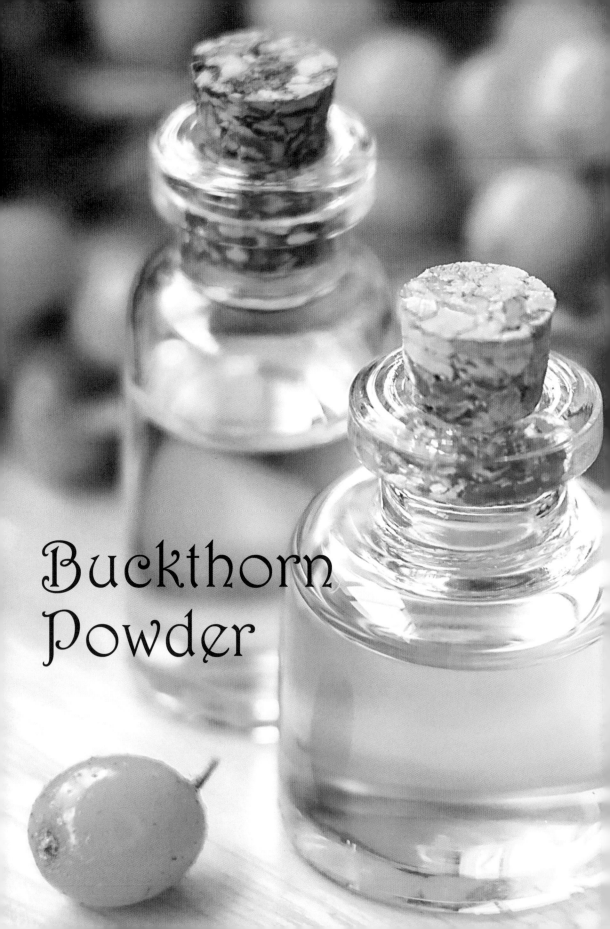

Buckthorn
Powder

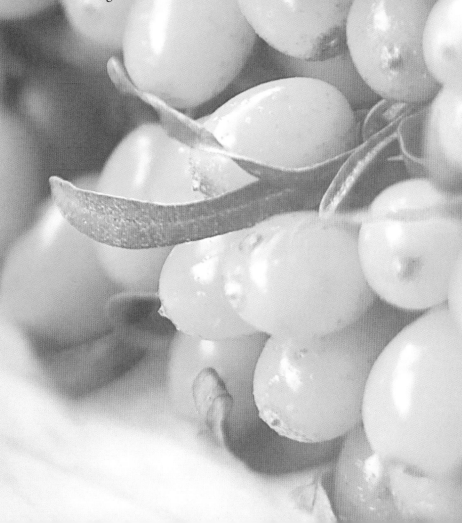

Sea buckthorn is a cold climate plant native to the mountains of China and Russia that produces berries throughout the winter. For thousands of years it has been used to treat a wide range of illnesses and is known as 'The holy fruit of the Himalayas.' It contains more than 60 antioxidants and is bursting with vitamin C. It also boasts B vitamins, folic acid, Vitamins E and K, a perfectly balanced ratio of essential fatty acids and 5-HT or serotonin, which is a neurotransmitter that regulates emotions. All these nutrients collectively boost heart health, the immune system, memory and concentration, the digestive system, circulation, skin health and it is also a fantastic anti-inflammatory.

To date, there have been more than 200 clinical and scientific studies advocating the amazing health benefits of what has been described as 'the most complete superfruit on the planet.' It has been shown to support growth, energy, slow down the ageing process, relieve sore joints and muscles, promote eye health and a healthy nervous system.

Uses – This powder has a naturally tangy flavour and so blends well with juices and smoothies. It is also good with yoghurt, porridge or puddings or even mixed with oil to make a delicious salad dressing.

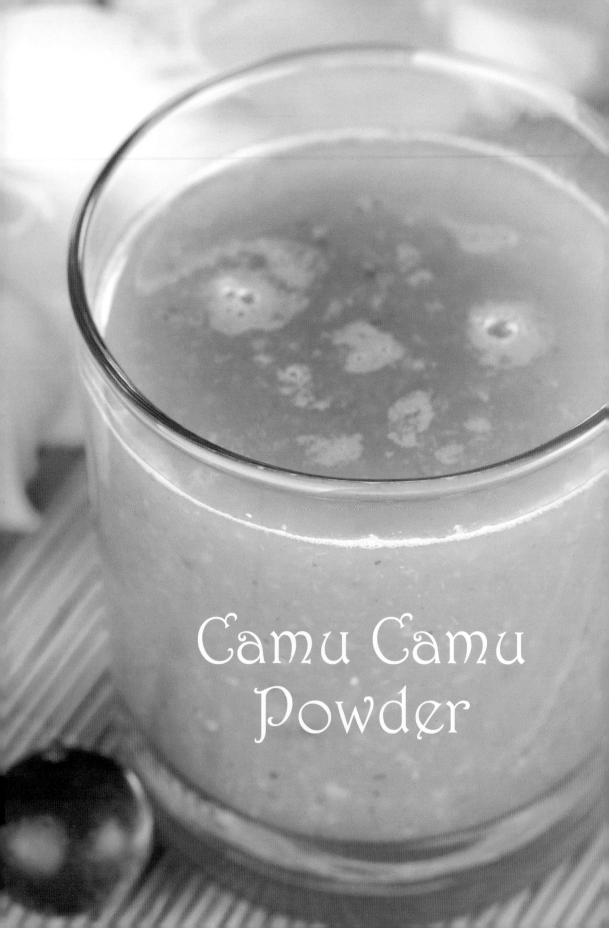

Camu Camu
Powder

Almost cherry like in appearance, camu camu is a fruit that grows in the South American rain forests of Venezuela, Brazil, Columbia and Peru. It is thought to be a natural sedative, a powerful natural treatment for depression and its high magnesium content is believed to have a positive impact on mood swings. It is also effective at treating diabetes, due to its high levels of antioxidants, and elagic acid which help to control blood sugar levels. It is highly antibacterial, helping to prevent infection, and it contains an amino acid called valine which aids a healthy nervous system. It is said to improve mental agility and boost the digestive system. Due to its high levels of vitamin C, it also boosts collagen production and reduces inflammation in the body.

Uses – Aside from adding it to juices and smoothies, try making camu camu lemonade or camu and mango frozen yoghurt. I love to add it to quinoa porridge which I make with quinoa flakes. How about making some lovely homemade energy balls by mixing with chia seed powder, hemp seeds, almond butter, dates, coconut oil, cacao and spirulina powder? Simply blend all the ingredients in a food processor, roll into balls and refrigerate.

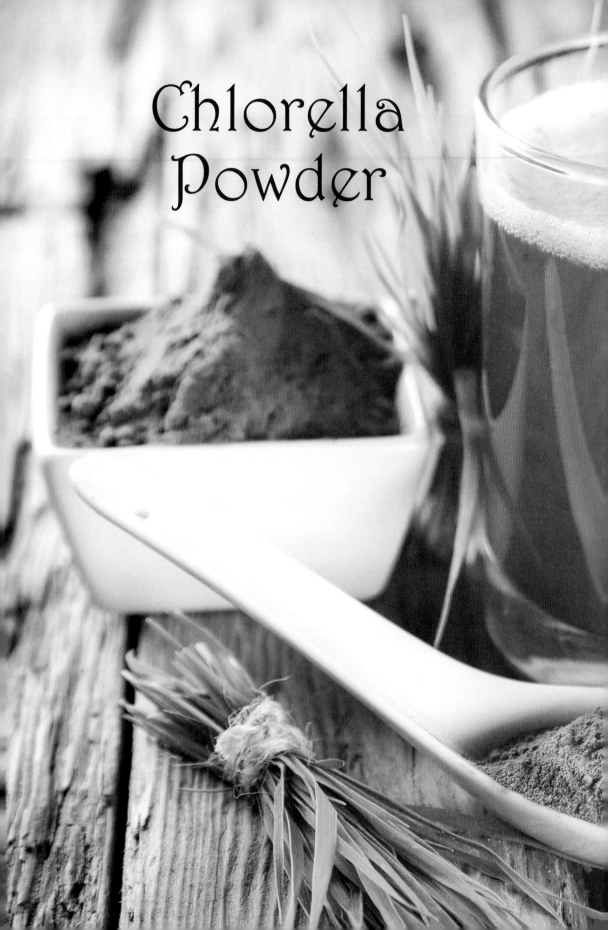

Chlorella
Powder

Chlorella is one of the most famous of the edible green algaes. It is a highly digestible vegetable protein and like wheatgrass, many of its health benefits come from its high chlorophyll content. It is rich in vitamins A, C, E and K and one of the few whole sources of vitamin D. It is believed to be one of the most nutrient dense foods in the world, and contains all the B vitamins and more beta carotene than carrots. Full of zinc, iron, calcium, magnesium and potassium, as well as essential fatty acids, makes chlorella an all-round immune boosting, energy enhancing, anti-inflammatory, anti-ageing, health and wellbeing super power food. It is a fantastic detoxifier and liver and intestine cleanser, it also helps to maintain a healthy PH level. Chlorella has been shown to balance oestrogen levels, reduce allergies, reduce blood pressure and cholesterol, and also balance blood sugar levels.

Uses – Like many superfood powders, especially the green ones, I find it easiest to add to raw juices and smoothies but you can also use it in vegetable soups and even jelly which is a great way to make it tasty for children.

Interesting Fact – Just one teaspoon of chlorella provides more nutrients than three whole servings of green, leafy vegetables.

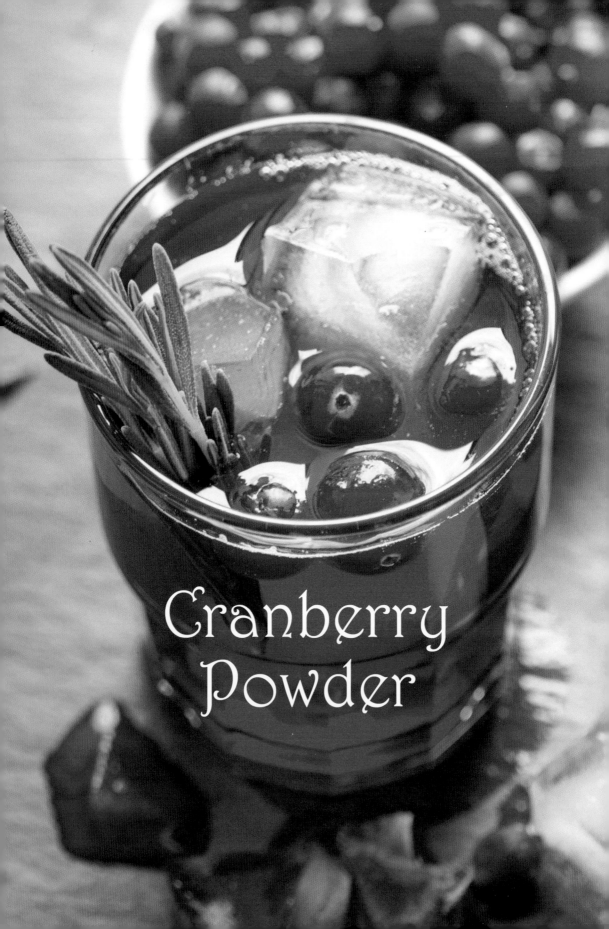

Cranberry
Powder

I have long been a fan of cranberry powder and other cranberry products (we have covered cranberries in the super fruits section separately) after suffering like many women from repeated bouts of cystitis. So I wanted to find not only an alternative to constant antibiotics, but prevention. Luckily I found exactly that with cranberry and I have used it to great effect for the past ten years. The cranberry is an evergreen shrub that grows in wet areas such as bogs. The plant has dark green leaves, pink flowers then the jewels of the crown, the dark red berries. Low in calories, virtually fat free, it contains no cholesterol, and is a super source of antioxidants as well as vitamin C & B, calcium, magnesium, iron, zinc and potassium. The proanthocyanidins in cranberry prevent bacteria from sticking to the bladder walls thus preventing infection and flushing them out through the body via the urine. It also makes the urine more acidic which is an environment in which it is difficult for bacteria to thrive and multiply.

Cranberries have also been shown to be tooth friendly by preventing the bacteria that causes plaque and tooth decay. It is effective in treating colds and flu symptoms as well as aiding the production of collagen in the body. As a natural anti-inflammatory and immune booster, they contain quinic acid, which has been shown to prevent the formation of kidney stones. Thought to aid weight loss by emulsifying fatty deposits in the body, this, along with the fibre content promotes a feeling of fullness for longer. It is thought the polyphenols (compounds) in cranberries may reduce the risk of heart disease and help to reduce blood pressure and there have been extremely positive results from studies showing that cranberries have actually slowed the growth rate of cancerous tumours. The combination of vitamins A and C make this a hair boosting food and taken daily could slow down the ageing process.

Uses – Well now we have established that cranberry most definitely should not be served only once a year with turkey, let's find out how versatile this super food really is. The powder can be added to almost anything both sweet and savoury, juices or foods. Why not have a go at cranberry and walnut bread or pear and cranberry jellies? Add to scones or make a maple and cranberry glaze for pork; and cranberry cookies and muffins are always popular – not just during the festive season! The juice is delicious and dried cranberries work well with everything.

Take note – Take care and consult your doctor if you are taking Warfarin or other heart medications as cranberry may interfere with this. Also get medical advice if you are a diabetic.

Goji Berry Powder

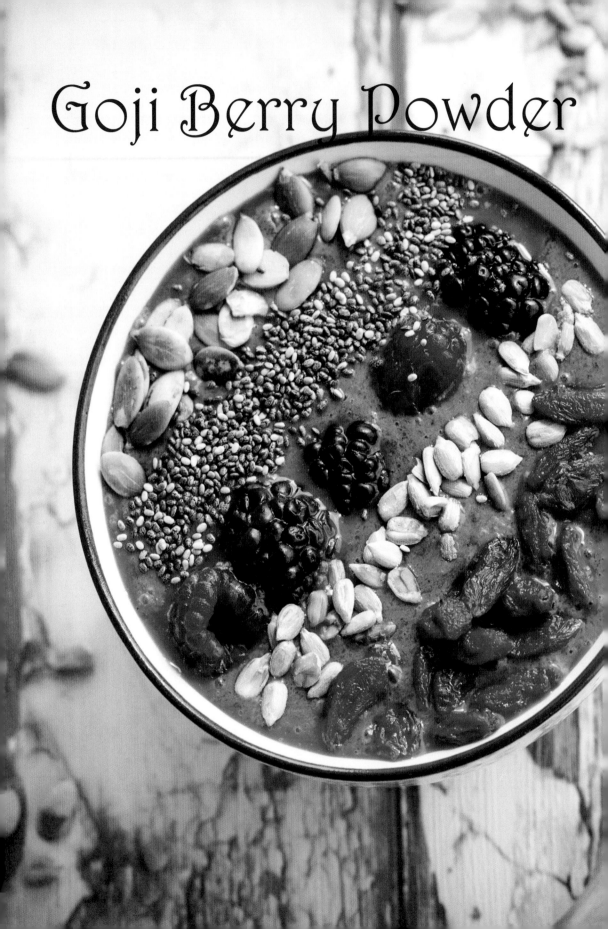

Goji is a bright orange-red berry native to China. It is a member of the nightshade plant family and has been used for thousands of years in Tibetan and Chinese cooking and medicine. These berries have the highest protein content of any fruit and boast all the essential amino acids. Bursting with vitamin C and fibre, calcium, zinc and selenium, they contain 15 times more iron than spinach. With their antibacterial, anti-inflammatory and anti-fungal properties, they are an excellent immune booster, low in calories, fat free and super rich in antioxidants which help our bodies fight off illness and disease. Overall, they promote a healthy digestive system, prevent constipation, may support healthy skin and eyes, and may boost eye health.

Uses – The berries themselves can be added to cereals or salads, and they can be made into juice which is extremely delicious and my son's absolute favourite, but the powder is incredibly versatile and can be added to any baking recipe for a super health boost as well as smoothies and juices. **Take note – You may suffer adverse reactions if you use goji whilst taking Warfarin or you have diabetes or use blood pressure medicines so please consult your doctor first.**

Interesting Fact – In Chinese medicine goji berries are believed to increase strength and longevity.

Lecuma Powder

Lecuma is a Peruvian fruit similar to an avocado with a hard, green exterior and a sweet, soft yellow fruit inside. It has been used for medicinal purposes for centuries. It has a sweet caramel like flavour which makes it perfect for baking recipes. In ancient times, it was used to support digestive health and to treat wounds, and more recent research has proven that it is beneficial for promoting healing of the skin. Rich in beta carotene, Vitamin B3, iron, zinc, calcium and protein, it is excellent for diabetics as it aids the regulation of blood sugars as well as being beneficial for heart health by helping to maintain healthy blood pressure levels. Lecuma is rich in antioxidants, and has antibacterial, antimicrobial (helps to kill harmful microorganisms) and anti-fungal properties as well as being thought to boost fertility and the immune system.

Uses – Lecuma powder is a naturally healthy sweetener, it is low in GI and low in calories yet bursting with nutrients and flavour. More like brown than white sugar, it can be used in a variety of recipes – just remember, for every tablespoon of sugar, use two of lecuma. This powder works well in smoothies, yoghurts, ice cream, muffins, cakes, porridge, pancakes and waffles. Lecuma ice cream is very popular in South America.

Interesting Fact – The lecuma fruit was deemed so important to the Incas that they even depicted it in their art. It was their symbol of fertility and creation, and was dubbed 'the gold of the Incas.'

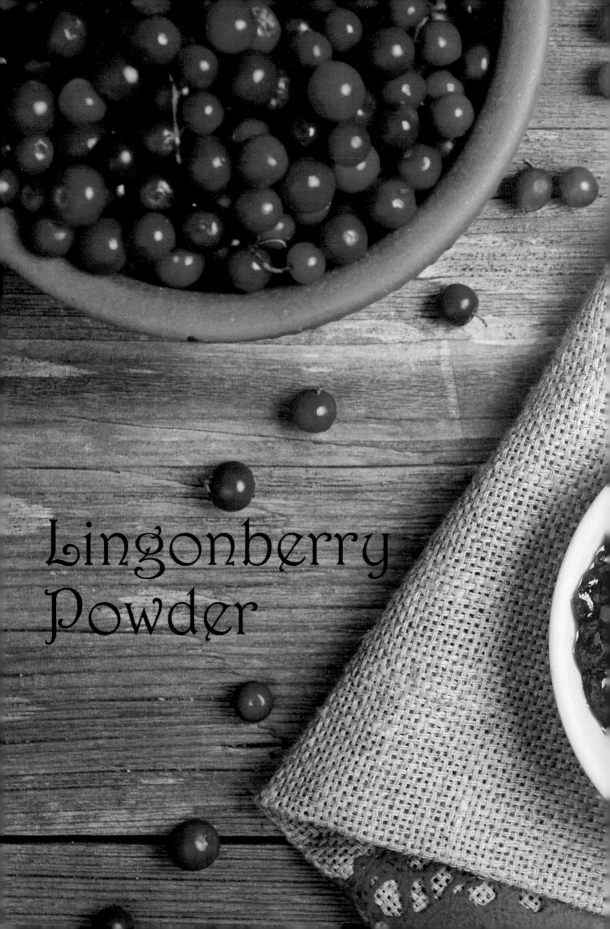

Lingonberry
Powder

Belonging to the same family as blueberries and cranberries, this little red fruit is native to the Arctic and the Subarctic. Bursting with antioxidants and containing more flavonoids than any other berry, they help to protect our bodies from cellular damage, disease and premature ageing. We have just talked about the benefits of using cranberry to prevent urinary tract infections, well lingonberries are another natural source of proanthocyanidins and are effective in the same way. It is thought that owing to the high level of polyphenols contained in lingonberries, they can help with weight loss and controlling blood sugar levels. They have also been shown to be a fantastic anti-inflammatory. High in fibre, and containing calcium, iron, potassium, sodium and magnesium as well as vitamins A, B, C, E and K, they promote a healthy digestive system and have a detoxifying effect on the body.

Uses – Add this deliciously tangy powder to your smoothies, juices, fruit and yoghurt. Try putting it in homemade rice pudding or a super healthy brownie or even a lingonberry cheesecake.

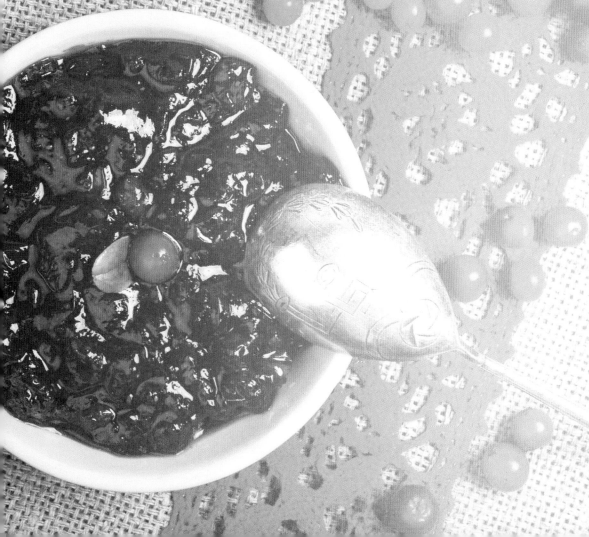

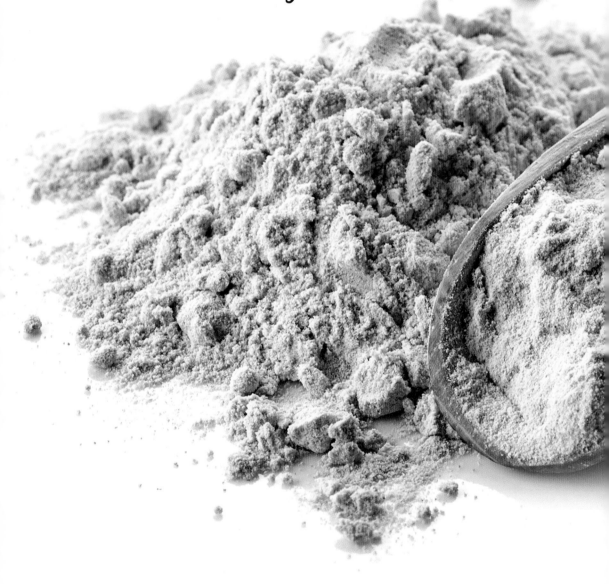

Maca Powder

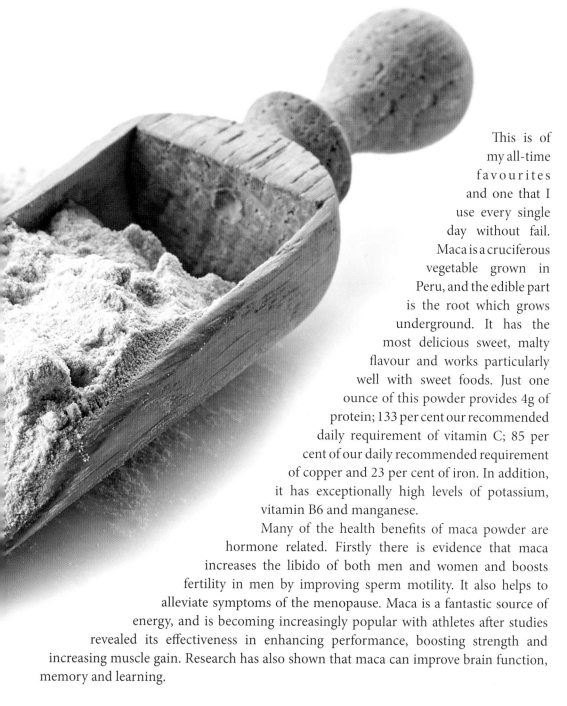

This is of my all-time favourites and one that I use every single day without fail. Maca is a cruciferous vegetable grown in Peru, and the edible part is the root which grows underground. It has the most delicious sweet, malty flavour and works particularly well with sweet foods. Just one ounce of this powder provides 4g of protein; 133 per cent our recommended daily requirement of vitamin C; 85 per cent of our daily recommended requirement of copper and 23 per cent of iron. In addition, it has exceptionally high levels of potassium, vitamin B6 and manganese.

Many of the health benefits of maca powder are hormone related. Firstly there is evidence that maca increases the libido of both men and women and boosts fertility in men by improving sperm motility. It also helps to alleviate symptoms of the menopause. Maca is a fantastic source of energy, and is becoming increasingly popular with athletes after studies revealed its effectiveness in enhancing performance, boosting strength and increasing muscle gain. Research has also shown that maca can improve brain function, memory and learning.

Uses – Whatever I decide to have for breakfast, I add maca, whether it's to smoothies, granola, porridge, fruit or yoghurt. It can also be used to make delicious truffles, pancakes, muffins or energy bars.

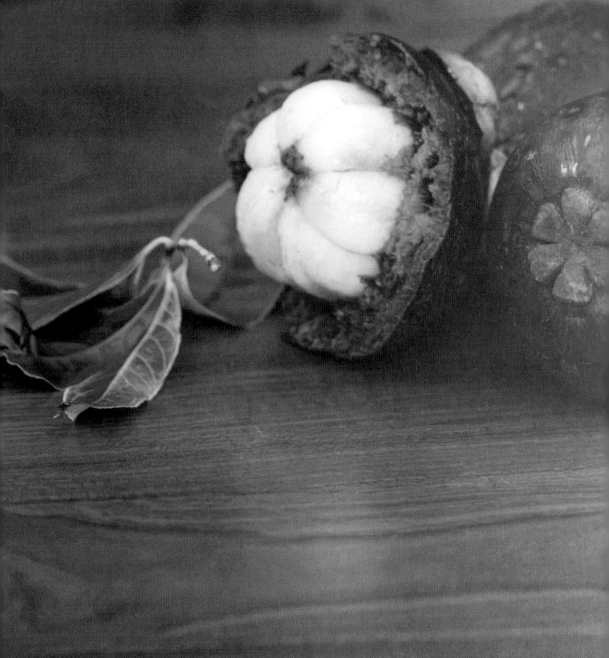

Mangosteen Powder

In South East Asia the mangosteen fruit has been used for medicinal purposes for centuries. It has been made into tea to treat everything from diarrhoea, gonorrhoea, thrush, urinary tract infections and menstrual problems as well as being made into a topical ointment to treat wounds, eczema, psoriasis and other skin problems. An exotic, tropical fruit, round and purple in colour on the outside with juicy white orange like segments on the inside, it tastes great in juices, smoothies, ice cream, toffee apples and pancakes.

Low in calories, fat and free from cholesterol, it is rich in fibre, vitamin C, B vitamins, copper, manganese, magnesium and potassium. Mangosteen is a fantastic immune booster and its antioxidants help to slow down the aging process and prevent damage from free radicals. It has been shown to dilate blood vessels, therefore increasing blood flow, and has also been shown to be useful in lowering cholesterol levels. Its excellent mineral content aids healthy blood pressure, and its antibacterial and anti-inflammatory properties make it extremely effective when used directly on wounds, acne, and eczema as well as both oily or dry skin. It has also been shown to regulate menstruation and is good for stomach problems.

Please note – It should be avoided if pregnant as it may be harmful to the foetus.

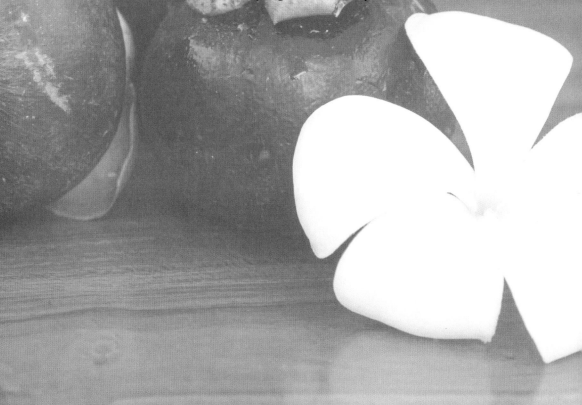

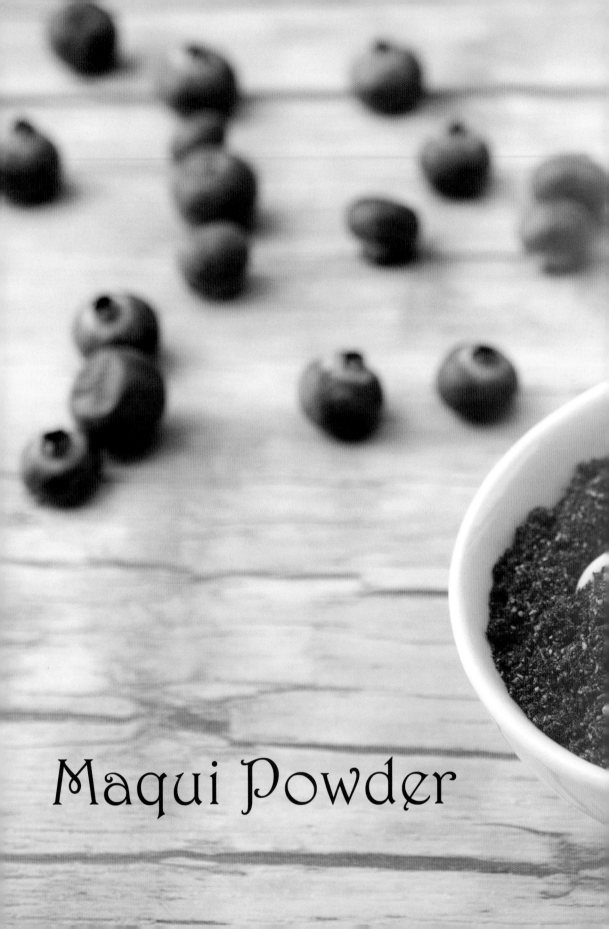

Maqui Powder

Maqui Banana Cacao Smoothie

Ingredients

2 teaspoons Maqui powder

2 teaspoons of Cacao powder

1 frozen banana

2 handfuls of frozen blueberries

1 tablespoon of almond of cashew
  nut butter

8oz of coconut milk, almond milk
  or soya milk

Blend all the ingredients together, adding more milk if required although I like my smoothies super thick and creamy.

You may top with additional blueberries, banana slices, grated cacao or sliced almonds – or a combination of them all.

Maqui berries are dark purple berries, similar in appearance to blueberries, and they grow in the rain forests of Argentina and Chile. They are super rich in antioxidants and also contain those wonderful anthocyanins (pigments), preventing free radical damage and reducing inflammation. They have been shown to increase insulin production and balance blood sugar levels therefore making them potentially useful for diabetes sufferers, and to kick start digestion, boost metabolism and provide an energy boost too. They are both antibacterial and antiviral and flush toxins out of the body. Maqui berries are also rich in vitamins and minerals especially potassium, calcium, iron and vitamin C, and provide an excellent boost to the immune system.

Uses – Simply delicious, so a welcome addition to many recipes but my favourites are maqui, banana and cacao smoothies, maqui berry and quinoa flake porridge, raw maqui berry fudge or oaty maqui berry energy bars.

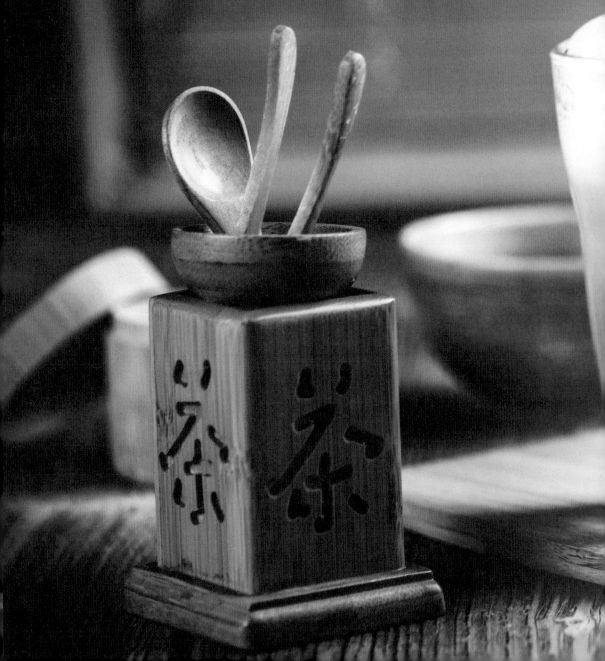

Matcha
Powder

Matcha is stoneground tea leaves which in powder form is rich in antioxidants, fibre, chlorophyll, vitamins, selenium, chromium, zinc and magnesium. It has been shown to boost the metabolism and burn calories, detoxify the whole body, lower cholesterol and blood sugars, relax both body and mind, and raise mood and concentration. Matcha contains a powerful antioxidant called catechin which is not found in other foods, and provides cancer fighting properties and protection against those damaging free radicals. Matcha has been shown to aid weight loss by boosting the metabolism and encouraging the body to burn fat whilst maintaining heart rate and blood pressure levels. It is rich in L-Theanine – the amino acid which promotes relaxation, countering stress and aiding memory. And I am certain you will remember all about chlorophyll, but just to remind you, it brings the body back to an alkaline state and is a powerful detoxifier. Not only will matcha give you an energy boost but it has also been proven to increase physical endurance. It is antibacterial and antiviral too.

Uses – It is very simple to make matcha tea but you are also able to add it to cooking, shakes and smoothies. Stir into scrambled eggs with spices and vegetables, sprinkle on granola, use to season vegetables or legumes, add to curries, mix with cream cheese for a twist on your regular bagel filling or blend with your favourite yogurt and freeze to make the healthiest ice lolly in the world!

Interesting Fact – Just one cup of matcha tea provides the nutritional equivalent of ten cups of regular green tea. Matcha powder contains 137 times more antioxidants than regular green tea.

Mesquite Powder

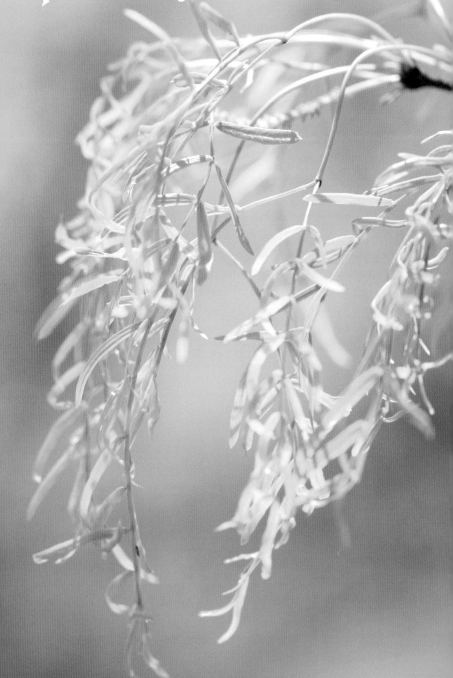

Mequite is native to South America and both the pods and the bark have been used for centuries for everything from making boats and furniture to flour. It is the beans inside the pods which are ground down to make the flour. The Mesquite tree grows slowly and needs very little water which is why they are often found in desserts. Both fat and cholesterol free, and full of soluble fibre boosting the digestive system and aiding the growth of friendly bacteria in the gut, mesquite is naturally gluten free and with its very low GI, is an excellent choice for diabetics. Rich in Omega-3 fatty acids and zinc, calcium, potassium, magnesium, copper and iron, it gives the immune system an extra boost, aids the reduction of blood pressure and boosting bone health.

Uses – Mequite wood is often used to smoke meats providing a lovely sweet flavour and mesquite is an ingredient often found in barbecue sauces. With its sweet, malty, caramel type flavour, mesquite makes a wonderful natural sweetener. The flours can be used in regular baking recipes of cookies, cakes, pancakes and breads, and the seeds can be roasted and added to soups, cereals and casseroles. Mesquite also makes lovely jams and jellies but mesquite powder can simply be used in regular tea, coffee and sweet beverages. Add to yoghurts, energy bars and juices and smoothies too. **Please note – the pods need to be cooked prior to consumption.**

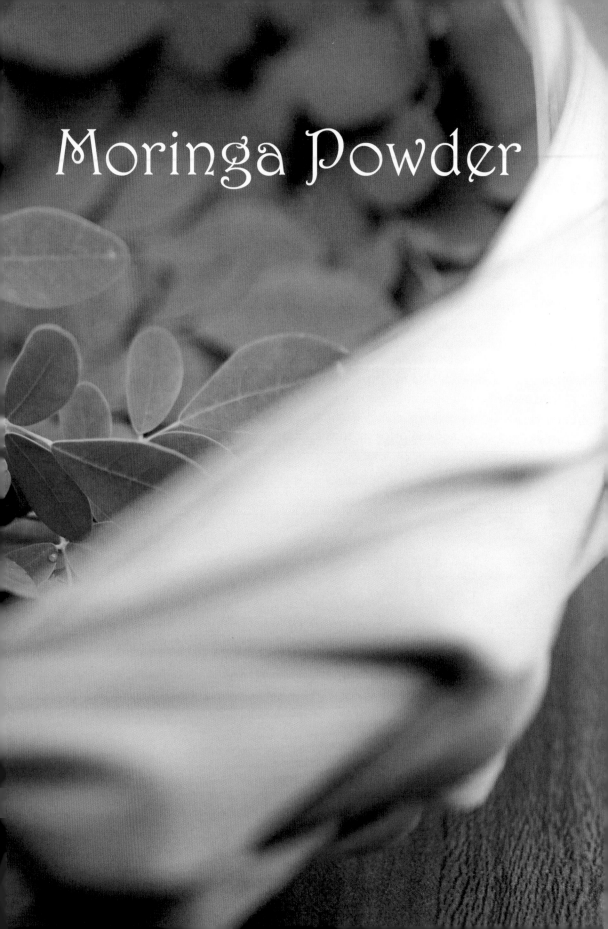

Moringa Powder

This powder comes from the moringa oleifera tree which is native to India, and has been revered for thousands of years for its amazing health benefits. It has been known as 'The Miracle Tree' for its healing properties. Recently scientists have been studying this tree to find out if it is it worthy of its reputation. Moringa contains more calcium than milk, more potassium than bananas, more vitamin A than carrots, more magnesium than eggs and more iron than spinach. It is a great boost for the digestive system and also thought to boost mood.

Full of protein, vitamins A, B and C as well as iron and magnesium, it is rich in antioxidants, in particular those that reduce blood pressure and regulate blood sugar levels. It has been shown to have anti-inflammatory properties and helps to lower cholesterol. As a complete protein, it supports bone health due to its calcium and magnesium content with one serving providing a huge 125 per cent of our daily recommended requirement of calcium.

Uses – You can actually buy moringa herbal tea, add the powder to juices or smoothies, sprinkle over cooked meats and fishes (after cooking to maintain full nutritional value), stir into soups or sprinkle over salads.

Interesting Fact – Almost every single part of the tree can be either eaten or used in herbal medicines but the leaves are the most nutritious part and the part most commonly used in India and Africa.

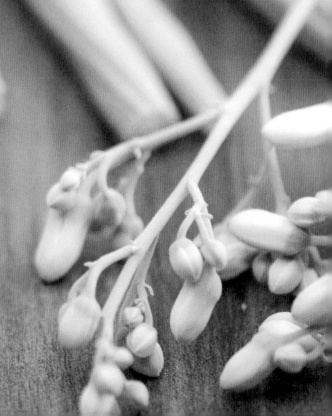

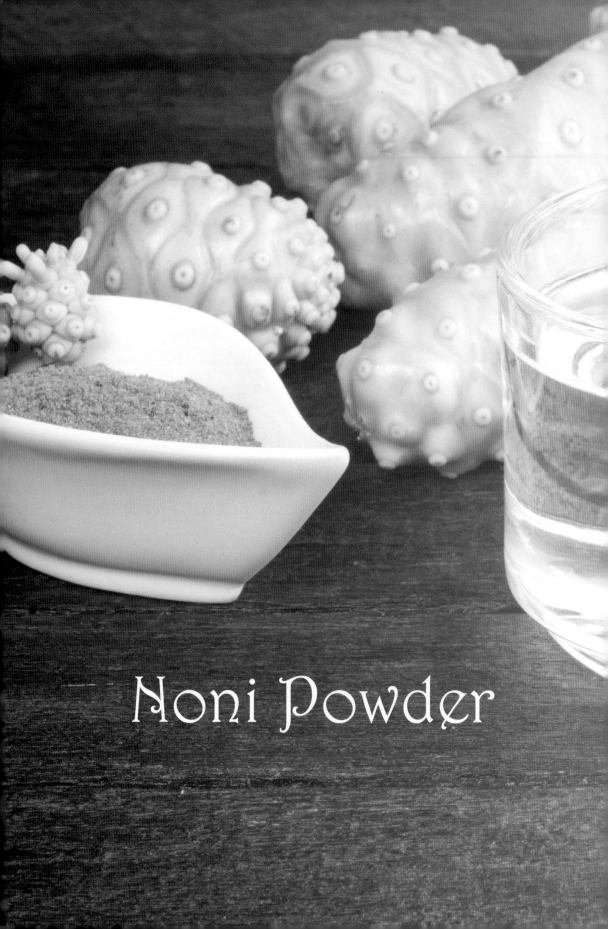

Noni Powder

Noni is a small evergreen tree which is found in the Pacific Islands, South East Asia, Australia and India. It has been known as ' The Painkiller Tree' as studies have shown it reduces pain as effectively as prescription painkillers. It is rich in fibre and so promotes a healthy digestive system and helps to soften stools. It also prevents LDL cholesterol from being absorbed. Noni contains the amino acid, tryptophan which has a tremendously relaxing effect on the body as it aids restful sleep and reducing stress. Furthermore, it is thought to reduce the symptoms of depression. In total, it boasts 17 amino acids, making it popular with athletes to aid recovery after training.

Noni helps boost the body's alkaline levels, and being rich in vitamin C, it is good for the immune system. It is antibacterial, helping to prevent infection, and its anti-inflammatory properties may reduce the symptoms of arthritis and other inflammatory diseases. It contains a compound called terpene which aids detoxification of the entire body.

Uses – Noni powder can be mixed in juice, milk or water but it also works well added to granola, porridge, yoghurt and even donuts, muffin and cookie mixture.

Interesting Fact – Historically noni was used to make red and yellow dye for clothing.

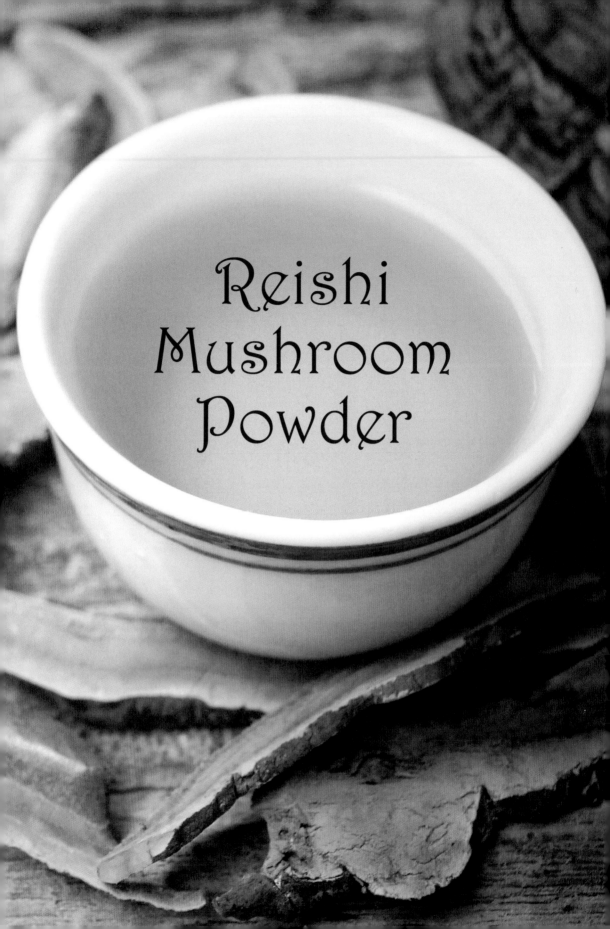

In ancient Eastern medicine the reishi was known as 'The king of immortality'. It really does seem hard to believe that this fungus – yes that's right, it is basically a fungus – has so many health benefits. Found growing on plum trees in the wild, reishi was originally reserved for use only by the royals. Over the years, there have been many sceptics of reishi, but extensive scientific research has now proven that it really is a super power. It is a fantastic immune booster and has even had amazing results in treating people suffering from AIDS and other immune disorders. Also it has shown to be effective in the treatment and prevention of cancer by slowing down the growth of tumours and boosting the immune system. Its glucan (a powerful molecule) content helps the immune cells bind to cancer cells and it is believed it actually reduces the number of cancer cells. In fact, in Japan it is recognized as a cancer treatment.

Reishi is a heart health super power too by lowering cholesterol, lowering blood pressure and even correcting arrhythmia, thus reducing the risk of coronary heart disease and stroke. Containing lanostan, which is a natural antihistamine, it reduces the risk and effects of allergies. It is also a powerful anti -inflammatory and pain reliever, and according to a study at The University of Texas Health Science Centre, it is equivalent to five milligrams of hydrocortisone. A 2013 study in food and chemical toxicology showed that reishi promoted liver cell regeneration and actually chemically reversed the damaged livers of mice. It has also been shown to support the production of nerve growth factor which in turn may beneficial for neurodegenerative disorders such as Alzheimer's disease or Huntington's disease. This mushroom has been used for many years for the prevention and treatment of viral infections, flu, fatigue, asthmas, bronchitis and nausea.

Uses – Now available in many forms from teas to tinctures to capsules but I find the powder the easiest and most versatile form. I often mix it with protein powder and add to my super food shakes and juices but it also adds nicely to soups and salads or stews and casseroles.

Spirulina Powder

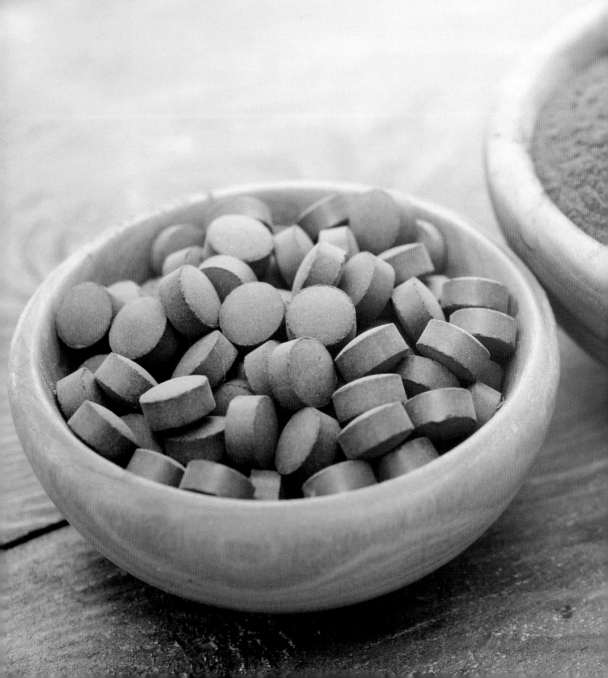

Spirulina is an algae that grows naturally in fresh warm lakes. This super food has so many health benefits that it is often recommended by doctors to treat a wide range of health conditions. It is a rich and complete food source containing more than a hundred differently nutrients – more than any other plant, herb or grain in the world. It contains magnesium, calcium, potassium, iron and zinc, the perfect B vitamin profile, several antioxidants and its bright green colour means it is also an excellent source of chlorophyll. Spirulina contains more protein than beef and fish (it has a 60 per cent content) and is said to promote heart health and boost the immune system. It has anti-cancer properties and boosts bones and possibly, the libido too. It helps to prevent depression and diabetes, slows ageing and boosts the metabolism. It detoxifies the body, balances PH levels as well as preventing fatigue.

Uses – Mix the powder into smoothies, juices, soups or add to homemade energy bars and granola. I make a delicious spirulina crunchy granola, but it can also be stirred into quinoa or added to wraps with avocado, sushi and salads – have fun with it!

Interesting Fact – Spirulina is one of the oldest life forms on earth and was responsible for producing oxygen in the earth's atmosphere billions of years ago, allowing life forms to develop.

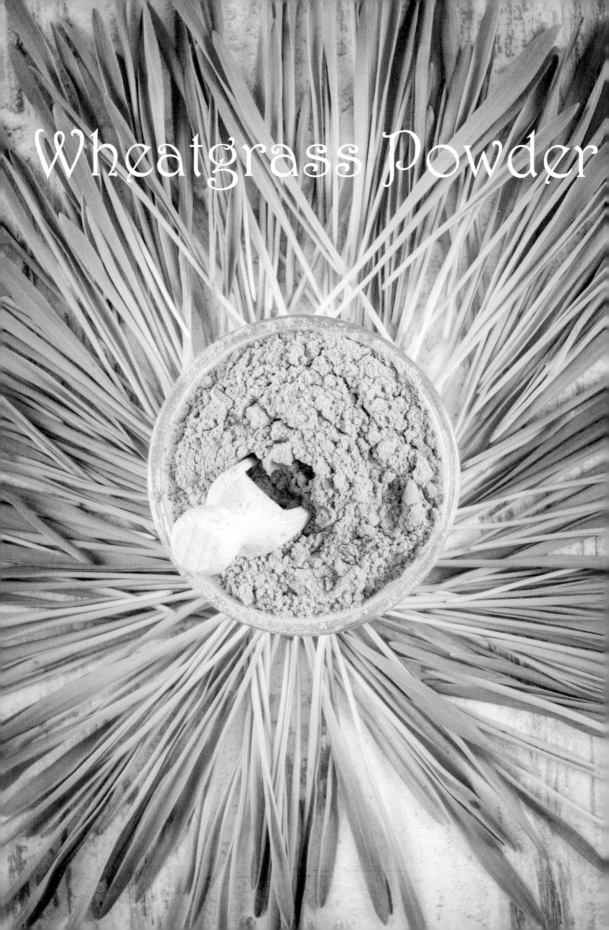

When I first began my quest to learn about nutrition and healing, wheatgrass was one of the first superfoods I came across. There was a lot of hype around it at the time and it was the word on the lips of every super foodie. I wanted to learn more about what it was, where it came from and what it could possibly do for me. The thing that first attracted me to wheatgrass was its name, as it is often referred to as 'liquid sunshine', due to its high content of chlorophyll (a green pigment that absorbs the sun's energy). Wheatgrass is the young grass of the wheat plant that is harvested when its nutrients are at a peak. It is a complete food and an excellent source of vitamins B, C, E and K as well as minerals calcium, iron, magnesium, phosphorous, sodium, potassium, sulphur and zinc. It also has an excellent amino acid profile.

So what does this all mean in terms of its health benefits? Well, one of its key strengths is to reduce the acidity levels in the body. An overly acidic system has been linked to a wide range of serious health conditions and unfortunately, stress, pollution and poor diet choices all contribute to an acidic system. Wheatgrass is very effective at bringing our PH level back (acid and alkaline measure) into balance. It has been shown to remove heavy metals from the system, and to reduce the symptoms of inflammatory ailments such as arthritis.

Wheatgrass is a fantastic blood builder so prevents anaemia, and as it is contains almost 50 per cent of protein, it is excellent for building and repairing muscles. It is rich in antioxidants too and extremely good for the intestines. A fantastic immune booster, it contains anti-cancer agents and compounds that help to lower blood pressure. It prevents the growth of bacteria, regulates blood sugar levels and has been shown to prevent cravings. It can even be put onto wounds to speed up healing and can help to clear bad breath.

Uses – You can buy or make wheatgrass juice but I keep the powder handy to add to my raw juices and smoothies. It can also be used to give pancakes an extra kick.

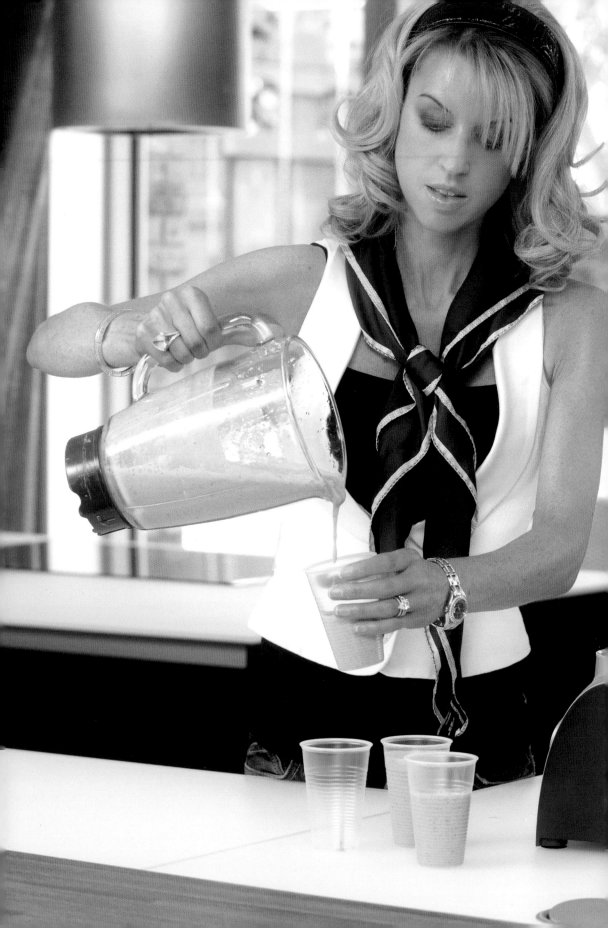

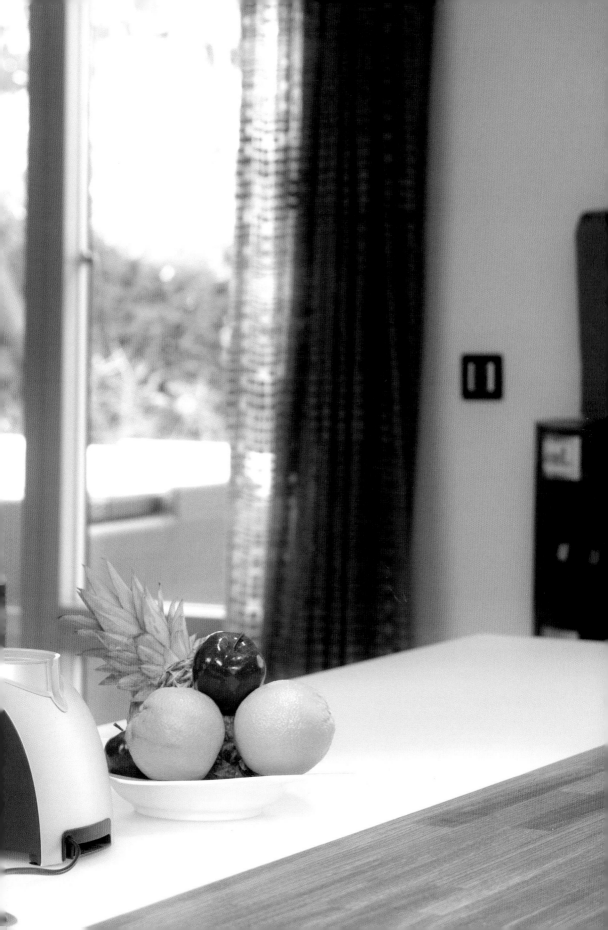

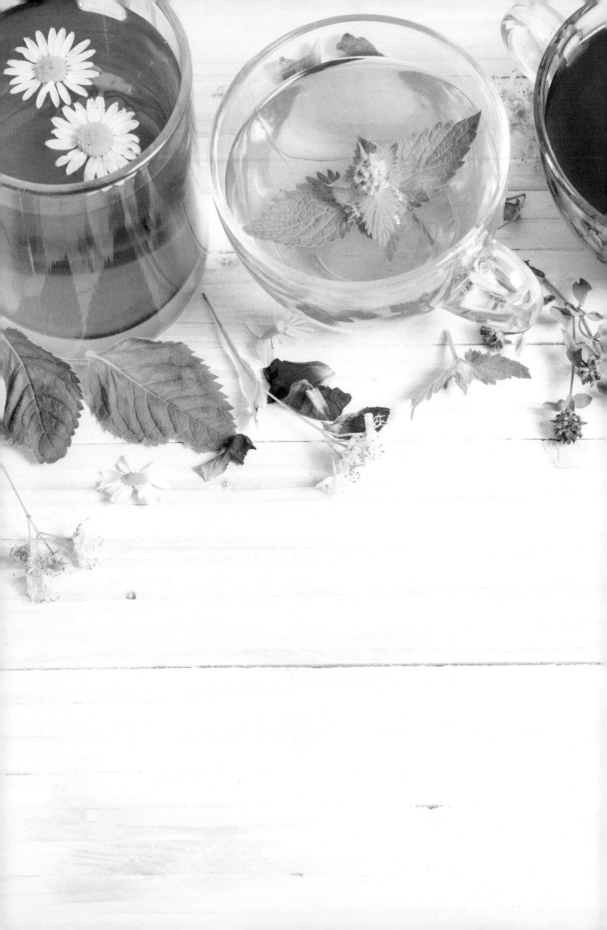

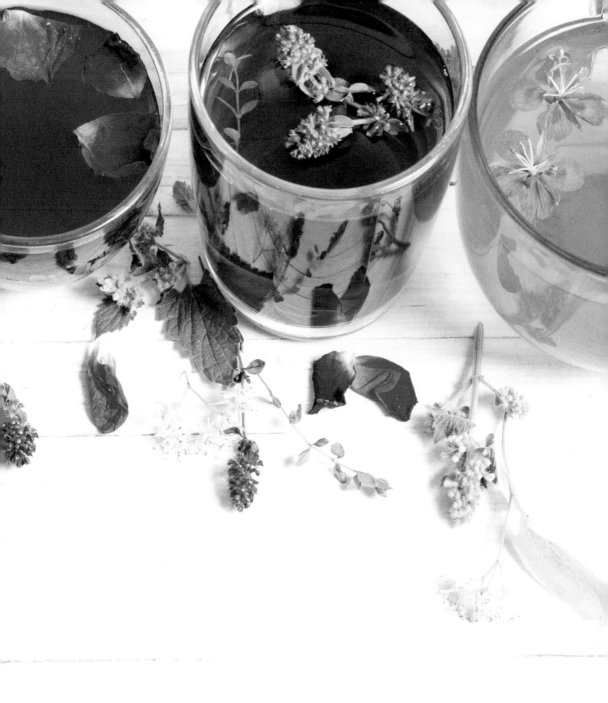

Super Teas

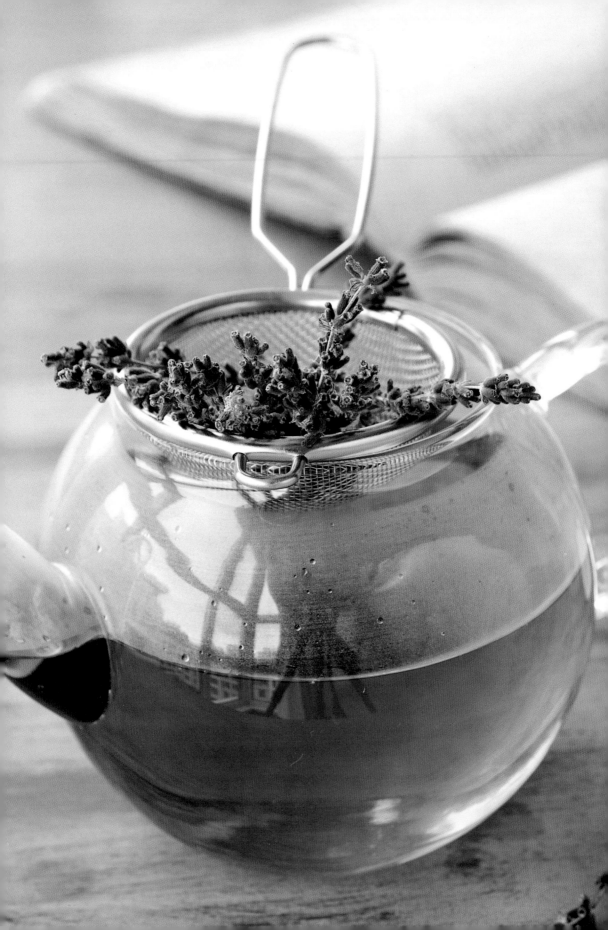

I think herbal teas are one of the most understated and undervalued drinks as most people simply don't realize just how beneficial they really are or what effects they can have. I currently live in Spain where they are not classed as teas but called 'infusions' which seems more apt. Herbal teas are not actually tea at all as to be classed as tea they would have to come from the Camellia Sinensis bush which is where all teas come from. They are infusions of leaves, bark, plants, seeds, flowers, herbs, spices and nuts that contain no caffeine and have a wide range of therapeutic and medicinal benefits. These benefits can range from simply relaxing, calming and relieving stress, detoxifying the body, calming the stomach, boosting energy, aiding restful sleep to promoting a healthy heart and boosting the immune system. Whilst the list of super teas is extremely long, those chosen for this book are some of my favourites that I have used for many years – but that is not to say there are not many more equally beneficial infusions available and I continue to experiment with new and exciting flavours and blends – and you should too.

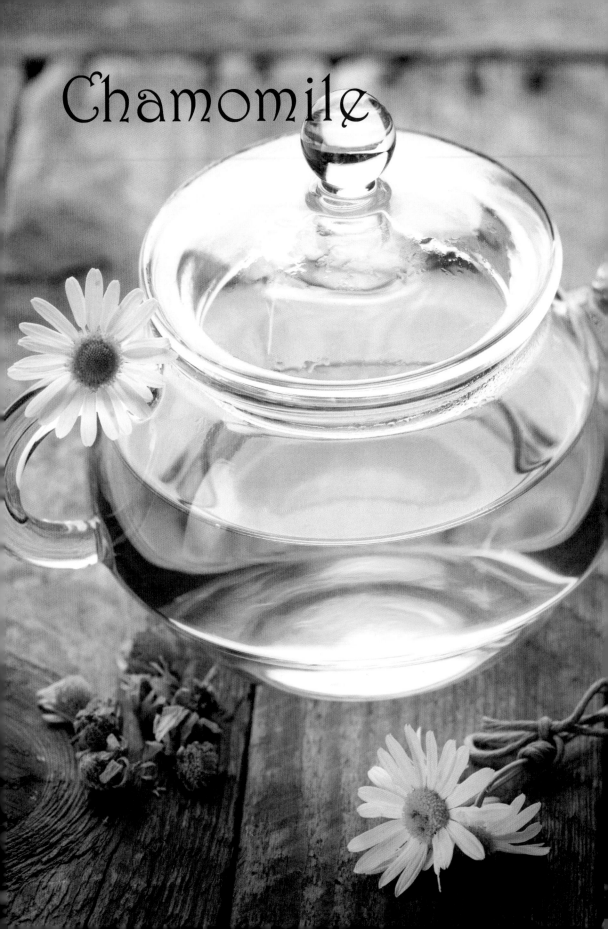

Chamomile

Chamomile is probably one of the most famous and readily available herbal teas and one of my favourites. It is an herb from the blooming plant of the Daisy family. Known as 'the calming tea' for its effects on the nervous system, chamomile is a fabulous bedtime drink. Its antibacterial properties make it good for treating or preventing colds. Chamomile has been shown to relax the stomach muscles thereby reducing the symptoms of IBS and upsets stomachs, as well as having positive effects on blood sugar levels making it another excellent choice for diabetics. But its benefits do not stop there, as it is also effective at promoting healing of all types of wounds, it promotes healthy skin and may also reduce menstrual cramps. Chamomile can be applied directly to the skin to ease eczema, rashes and allergies, or placed onto the eyes to sooth sore or tired eyes and to reduce under eye bags and circles. It is also a natural cleanser for the skin, hair or scalp. My favourite way to drink this cup of calmness is with boiling water (left for five minutes) and a little manuka honey added to boost both sweetness and health benefits.

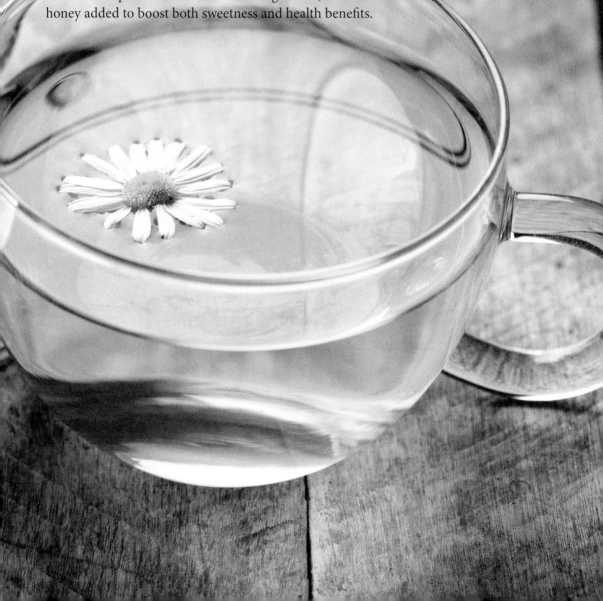

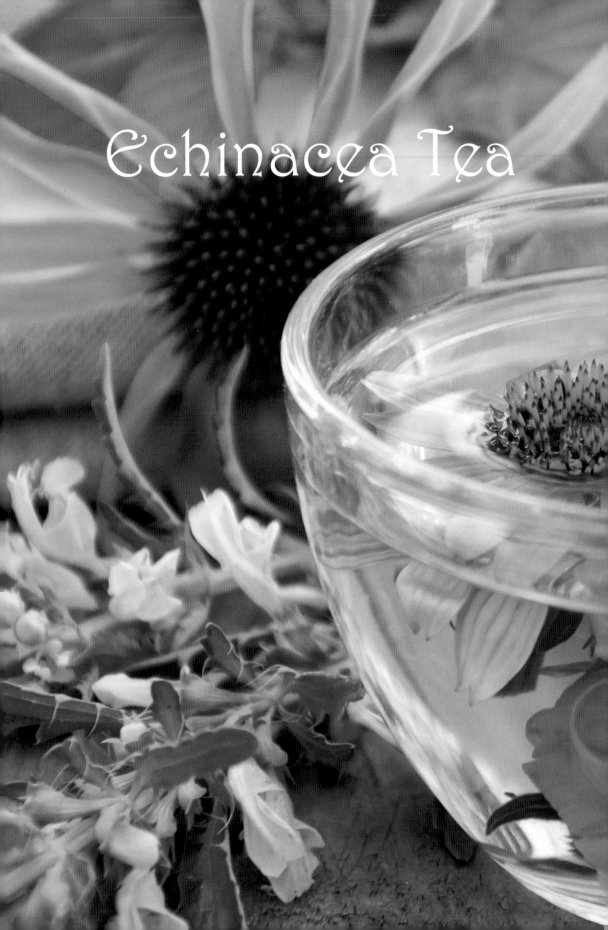
Echinacea Tea

I am guessing that the majority of you have heard the rumour that echinacea is useful for preventing and treating colds – well the University of Maryland Medical Centre proved this rumour to be true with research revealing that echinacea can reduce the risk of catching a cold by a whopping 58 per cent. This herb is native to the American Indians who uncovered it around 400 years ago, with the roots, leaves and flowers all used, it has proven itself to be very powerful indeed. Able to increase the production of white blood cells, it is an excellent immune booster as well as containing natural antiseptic properties.

Echinacea is a fantastic source of vitamins and minerals and contains calcium, iron, selenium, magnesium and zinc. Its phytochemical content makes it an anti-cancer herb and it has also been shown to be effective at treating skin conditions both internally and externally such as psoriasis and eczema. It is known for being a natural painkiller and a laxative, preventing constipation and the removal of toxins and waste from the body. Finally it is thought to be extremely calming to the body and mind, and therefore may be useful in treating anxiety and stress-related illnesses. The tea can be made using the leaves but it is thought that tea made with the tincture is even more beneficial.

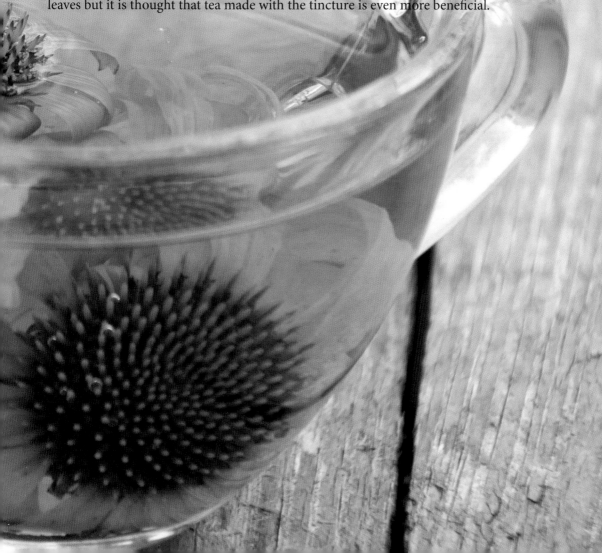

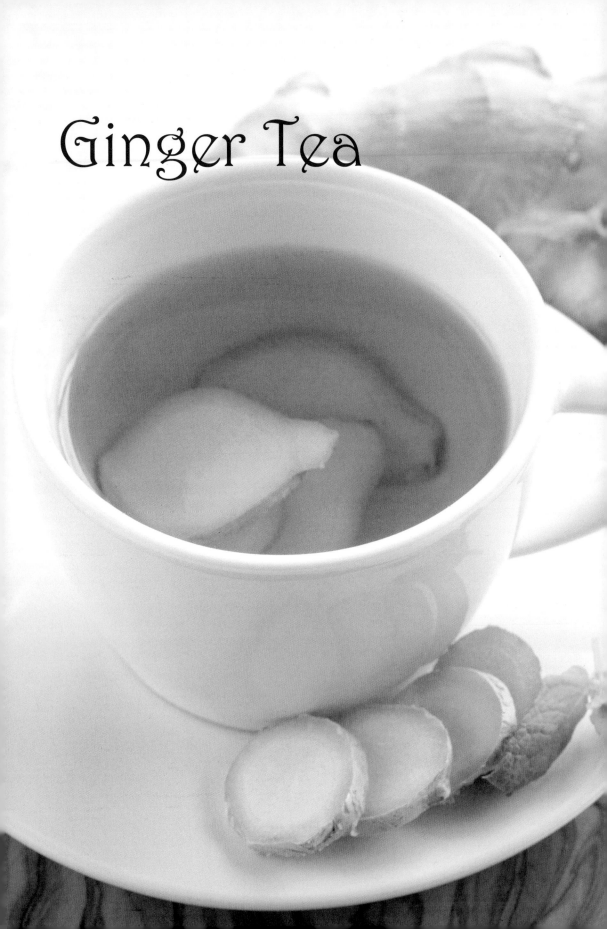

Ginger Tea

For over two thousand years ginger has been used for its medicinal purposes and it is known to be one of the most nutritious spices in the world. The list of health benefits is substantial and I am a huge fan – in fact, I put so much raw ginger in my super smoothies that I have to make a separate batch for my children as they complain that mine are so hot they burn their throats. Ginger has an excellent reputation for calming the stomach and eases the symptoms of IBS, motion sickness, morning sickness or heartburn. It has a fantastic relaxing effect on the intestines, relieves gas and has also been shown to prevent acid from regurgitating back into the oesophagus.

Ginger also balances blood sugar levels, and has a suppressive effect on the appetite and so may be useful in aiding weight loss. It increases blood flow and circulation, making it a wonderful winter warming drink. As a powerful natural anti-inflammatory, it reduces the symptoms associated with arthritis and asthma and helps to open the airways. Ginger has been shown to flush out toxins and to boost the immune system and the libido. It contains anti- cancer properties in particular a compound known as 6-gingerol which has antibacterial, anti-inflammatory and anti-tumour properties. Not only is ginger a fantastic cancer preventer, it actively destroys cancer cells and has been shown to be effective in reducing the side effects of the cancer drugs and so is beneficial for those receiving cancer treatment too. Ginger tea is absolutely delicious, warming and nourishing. I like it alone but it is popular to add lemon or honey to taste.

Interesting Fact – Chinese medicine believes that ginger restores yang – or hot energy.

Ginseng Tea

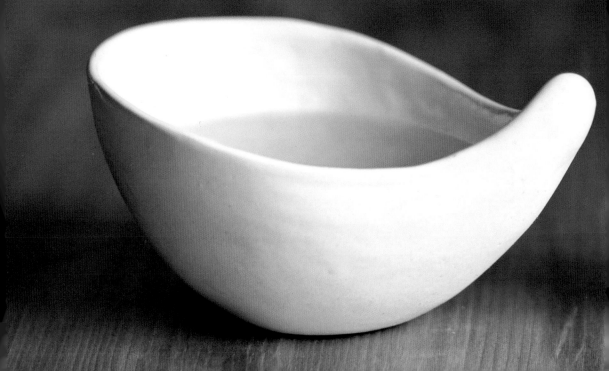

Ginseng originated in China and has been in use for more than five thousand years. It was once deemed to be so valuable that it was exchanged for silk and even gold! The tea is made from the fleshy root of the ginseng plant. Ginseng is thought to provide energy, boost concentration and aiding weight loss by supressing the appetite and boosting the metabolism. It has also been shown to reduce the symptoms associated with menstruation. Rich in anti- cancer properties, it has been proved to improve blood sugar levels. It is best left in boiling water for between five and 15 minutes, and should be drunk three to four times a day.

Take note – Consumption of ginseng may interact with blood thinning and blood pressure medications and anti- depressants so always consult your doctor first. It has also been shown to reduce the heart rate and therefore should also be avoided by anyone with a heart condition. It is not suitable for pregnant or breastfeeding women or those with uterine problems.

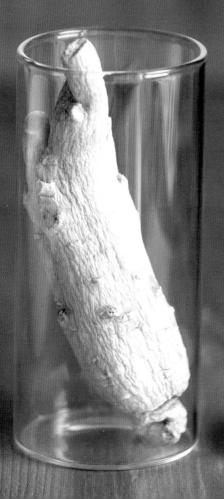

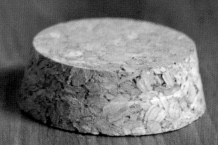

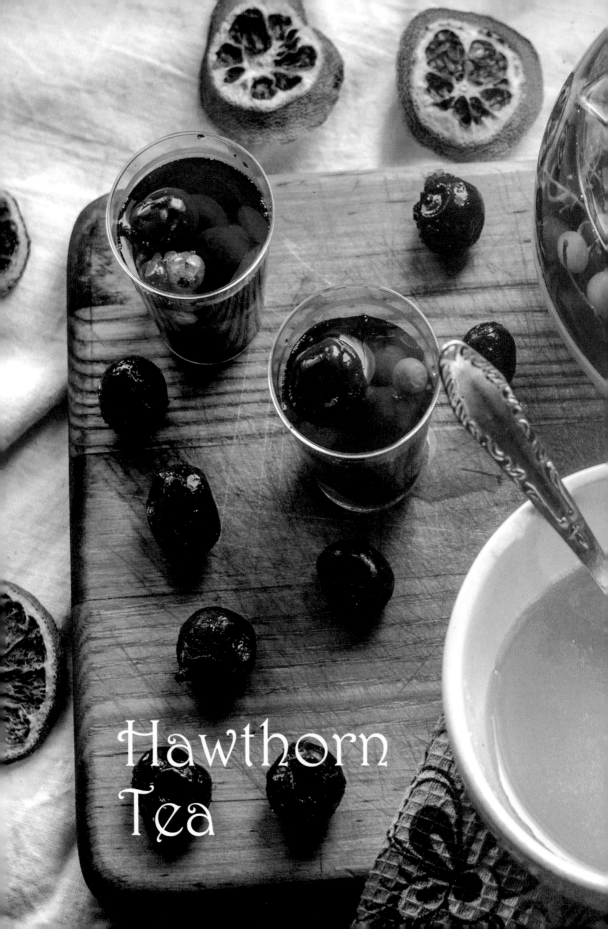

Hawthorn
Tea

Grown in many parts of Europe, the hawthorn berries, leaves and flowers can be used to make tea. My interest in this tea stemmed from its heart health benefits. Whilst some people inherit beauty or brains, my family decided to pass down a gene that unfortunately leads to heart disease and many of my family members have suffered or are suffering from heart related conditions. But in hawthorn, we have found a wonderful heart health tonic as it increases the blood supply and oxygen to the heart increasing overall circulation. It has also been shown to be effective in strengthening the arteries, preventing blockages and inflammation as well as maintaining healthy blood pressure and cholesterol. However, its abilities do not stop there. It is rich in vitamins and minerals (especially vitamin C) as well as antioxidants, preventing damage from free radicals. It provides an excellent boost to the immune system as well as being a natural sedative, calming nerves and tension and promoting restful sleep. Best left to steep for 10 minutes in boiling water, it does have a slightly tart flavour and so may be sweetened with a little honey or even sprinkled with cinnamon.

Interesting Fact – Did you know that Hawthorn is used to dress the Queens table at Christmas?

Lavender Tea

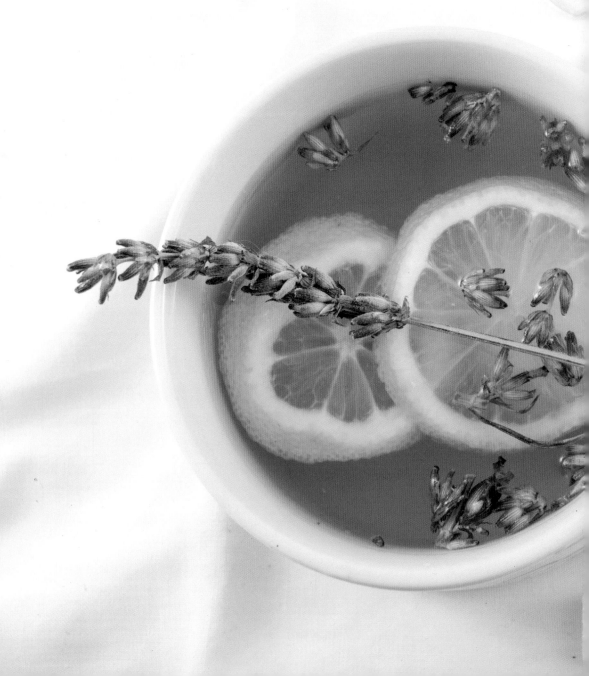

Lavender brings back memories of my grandmother who often had bags of lavender in her drawers. Little did I know at the time just how wonderful these little purple flowers really are. The Latin name for lavender is 'lavare' which means 'to wash' based on its clean aroma. If using fresh lavender buds, place into a tea ball and leave in boiling water for ten minutes prior to drinking.

Best known for promoting relaxation and preventing anxiety, lavender is also highly antispasmodic, helping to relax the intestines and providing relief from stomach cramps and nausea. Also now known to be an excellent pain reliever, it is especially effective for joint, muscle and menstrual pain. Highly antibacterial, lavender can prevent infection and support the immune system and it also thought to help treat depression, and has been used for coughs and respiratory problems.

Interesting Fact – Did you know that up until the end of the First World War, lavender was used to treat the wounds of the soldiers?

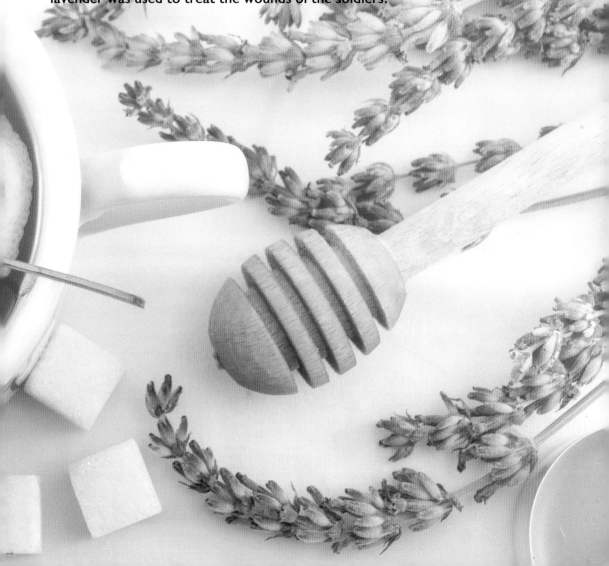

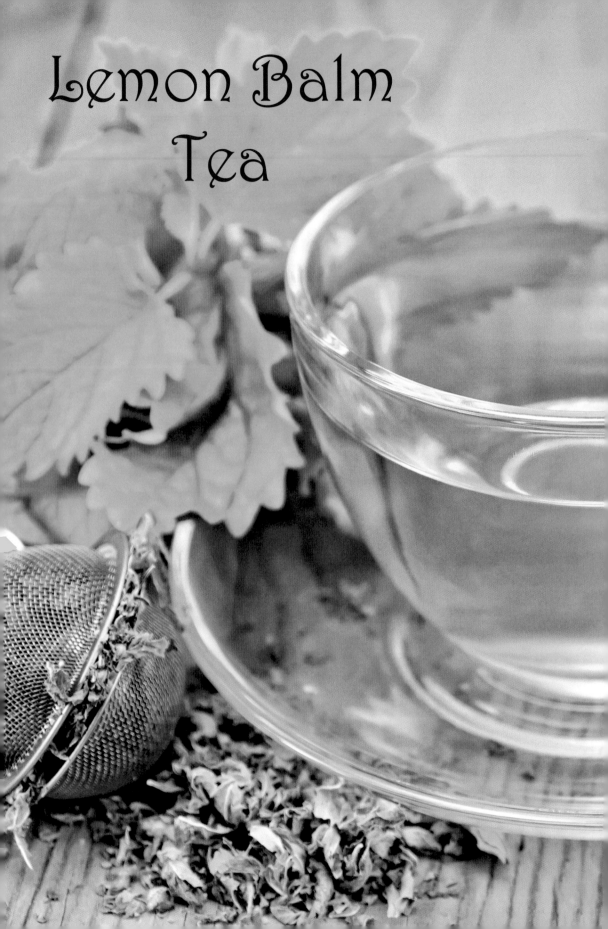

Lemon Balm
Tea

Lemon balm is a herb, and is actually part of the mint family. It has a tremendously relaxing effect on the body and has been proven to be useful in the treatment of insomnia, to reduce anxiety and support the nervous system. It is bursting with antioxidants, providing an immune boost and helping to prevent premature ageing. It also soothes the digestive system and intestines as well as increasing alertness and boosting mood. Studies have shown that it increases memory and although in its early stages, it is showing positive effects on patients suffering from Alzheimer's disease. It is thought to maintain normal blood sugar levels and to also aid the liver in the removal of toxins from the body. Lemon balm is commonly used in cosmetics and is extremely effective when applied to skin conditions and cold sores as it contains compounds that help to fight the herpes virus.

Take note – Lemon balm may interact with thyroid and HIV drugs so seek advice from your doctor before use.

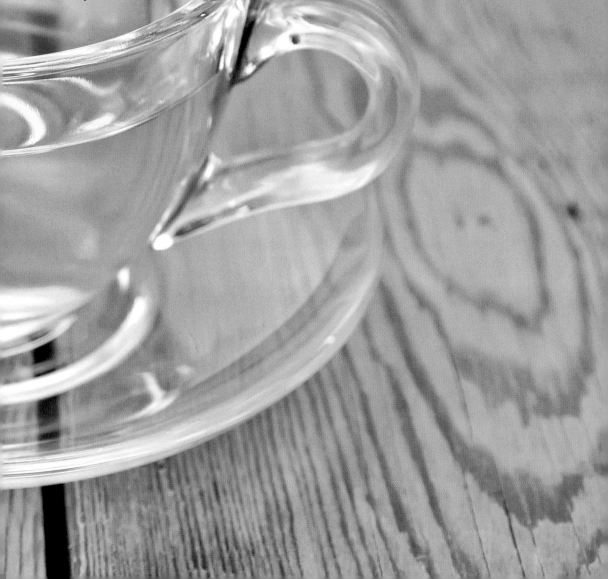

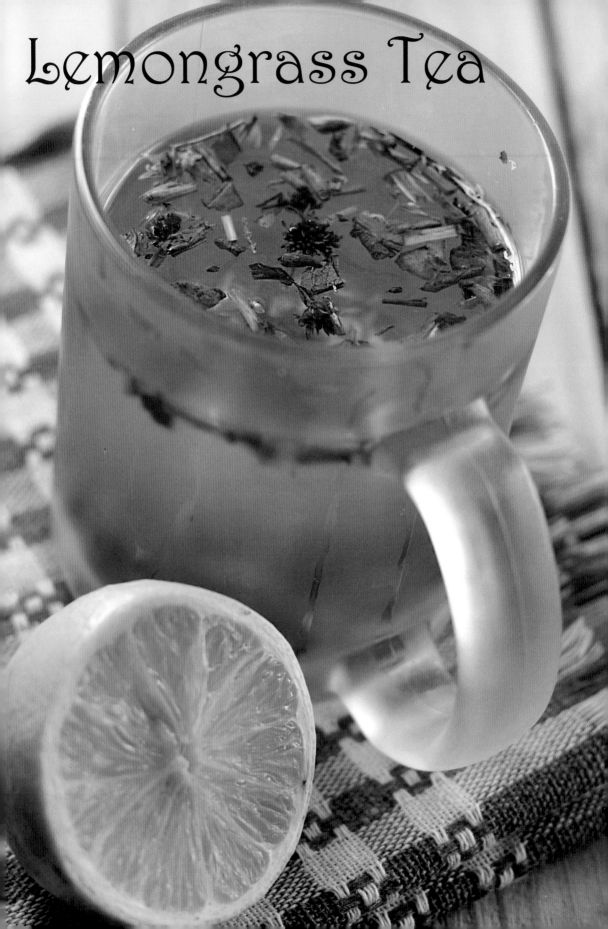

Lemongrass Tea

Not surprisingly, the lemongrass plant has grass like leaves with a lemony fragrance. It is native to India and the tropical regions of Asia and the plant stands about three metres in height. It is antibacterial, antifungal and antimicrobial, rich in vitamin A, B vitamins and vitamin C as well as the minerals magnesium, potassium, copper, calcium, iron and zinc. Being full of antioxidants makes it good for fighting off those free radicals. It also contains a specific component called citral which can prevent the growth and production of cancer cells. Lemongrass has also been shown to help maintain healthy cholesterol levels as well as flushing toxins and waste out of the body thus aiding the liver and kidneys and promoting a healthy digestive system. It is extremely calming and thought to be effective in treating insomnia as well as giving the metabolism a kick start and helping the body to burn fat.

Uses – Lemongrass has been used for years in various dishes especially Thai food, curries and sauces, and the tea can be enjoyed both hot and cold as a bedtime drink.

Take note – It is not suitable for pregnant or breastfeeding mothers.

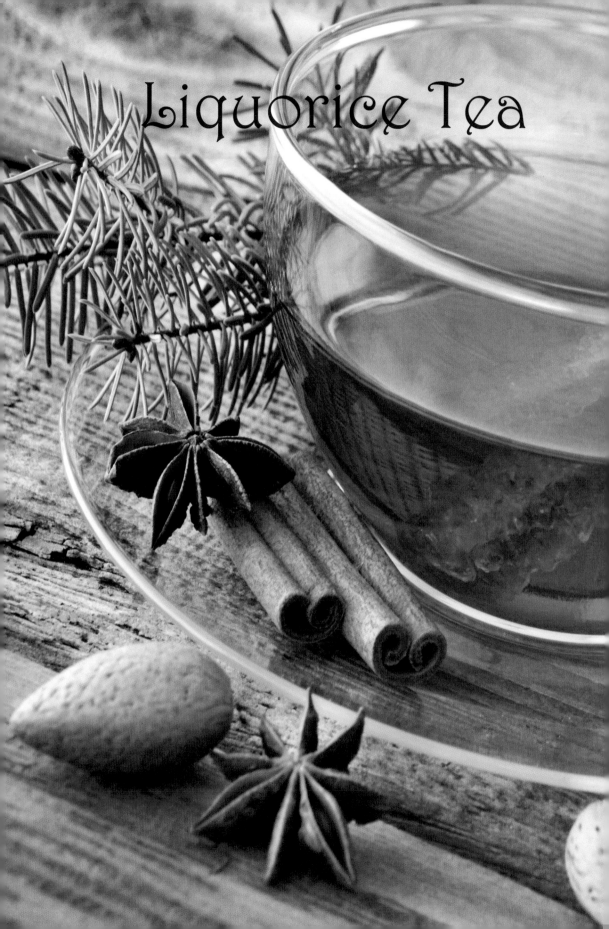

Liquorice Tea

Liquorice tea is becoming extremely popular in both Middle Eastern and European countries not just for its aromatic flavour but for its increasing reputation as a true superfood. Originally discovered in Asia, the liquorice comes from the plant's root which is dried out and then made into tea, capsules or liquid extracts. The root is the most used herb in Chinese medicine. Studies have shown that people who consume liquorice regularly have a decrease in body fat and it has also been shown to be fantastic for the liver. Good for the respiratory system too, it loosens the mucus and soothes the throat and sinuses. A study published in the journal *Evidence-Based Complementary and Alternative Medicine* showed that liquorice was a natural remedy for heartburn, nausea, stomach cramps and indigestion, and further studies revealed that its anti-inflammatory properties make it a powerful remedy for ulcers.

This wonderful herb actually came across my radar at an extremely difficult time in my life, after the birth of my daughter. She was extremely unwell for a long time as was I. With a one-year-old at home, a new born in intensive care and my husband working away, I suffered prolonged periods of extreme stress which finally resulted in adrenal fatigue. I didn't want to medicate to help me cope and then I found liquorice, which as I discovered is fantastic at regulating cortisol (the stress hormone), thus providing welcome relief for the adrenal glands. I personally have used it for many years with great success and now recommend it to so many people. But it´s health benefits do not end there as its highly antiviral properties boost our immune systems and the use of liquorice has been shown to be more effective than HRT at treating the hot flushes, often associated with the menopause, as well as being useful for treating infertility and menstrual problems.

Take note – Liquorice should be avoided if pregnant, and not be used for babies or nursing mothers. It may interact with prescription medicines so take advice from your doctor before using.

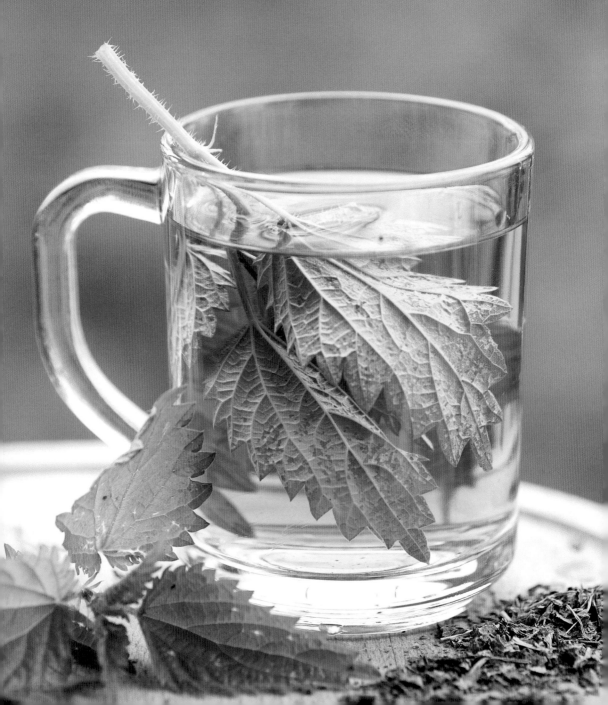

Nettle Tea

We have gone full circle with nettles; from our parents advising us to stay away from them as children, and now as adults, we are being advised to consume them! Nettle tea contains 17 essential vitamins and minerals as well as fatty acids and phytochemicals. It is also rich in lycopene which is known to fight off cancer cells. The root and leaves of the nettle plant contain chemical compounds that are biologically active. Consuming nettle tea has been shown to be effective in treating and preventing allergies and it has also been shown to stimulate the lymphatic and digestive systems thus aiding the detoxification of the body. It may help to break down stones in the liver or gall bladder as well as preventing urinary tract infections and water retention. Research has also shown it to be effective at treating gout, arthritis, muscle pain and other inflammatory conditions. Beneficial for both bone health and the respiratory system, it is antibacterial and also effective in treating PMT symptoms such as cramping and bloating. For the full benefits of nettle tea, pour boiling water over the dried leaves and leave for fifteen to twenty minutes before drinking – allowing time to deactivate the stingers!

Take note – Nettle tea may interfere with anti-depressants, anti-anxiety or blood pressure medication, so seek advice from your doctor before using.

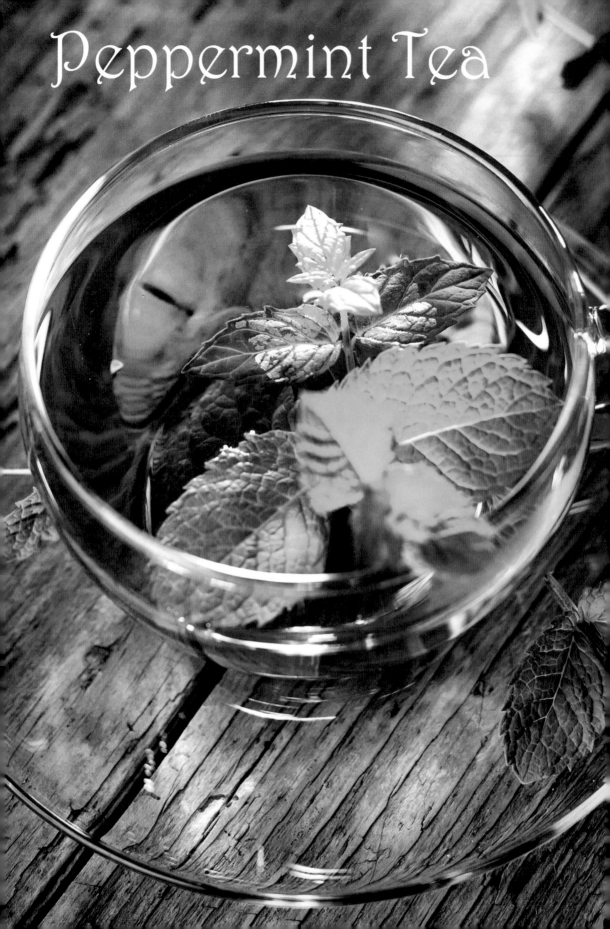

Peppermint Tea

Now this is my go to item for any stomach upsets and it has been used for centuries for its medicinal properties. This tea is now recommended by both natural therapists and doctors for a wide range of health conditions. Peppermint contains the active ingredient menthol which has an antispasmodic effect which is why it is so effective in treating stomach cramps, upsets and IBS. It is also antibacterial, antiseptic and antimicrobial so helps to fight infections and is a natural decongestant. It has been shown to promote alertness and concentration, to reduce menstrual cramps as well as relieving stress and balancing hormones. Peppermint can be consumed in two ways, with the dried leaves in the bags or simply with fresh mint through a tea strainer or fresh mint which I adore. Simply add some fresh mint leaves to a pot, add boiling water and leave for five to ten minutes – my perfect after dinner drink!

Interesting Fact – Did you know that the smell alone of peppermint tea can relieve the symptoms of colds and headaches?

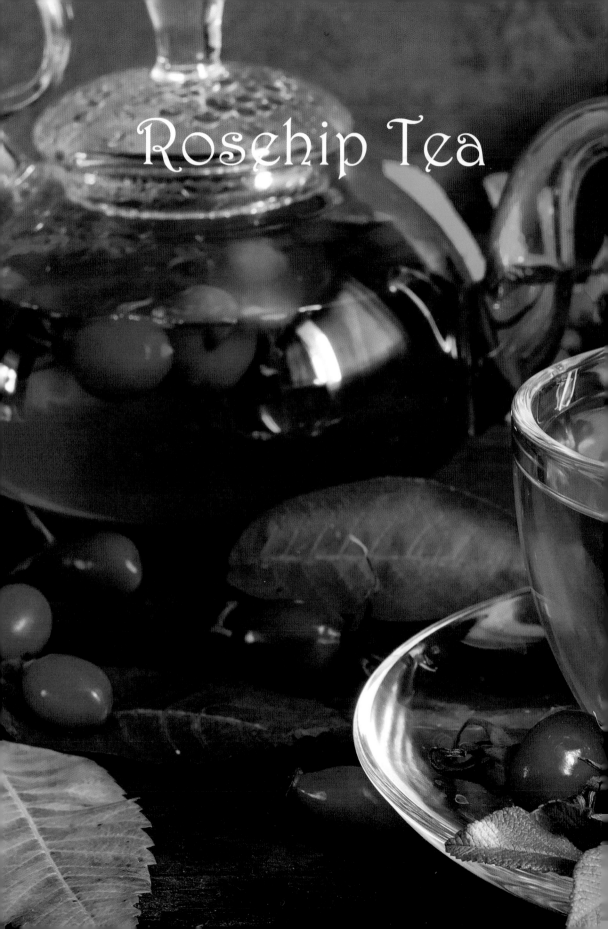

Rosehip Tea

Rosehip is actually the fruit of the rose plant which grows up to a staggering ten feet tall and produces the most fragrant flowers. Similar in shape and size to cherries – the seed must not be eaten, although it can be dried along with the rosehips for medicinal use. Rich in vitamins, calcium, iron, selenium and manganese, it is an immune boosting drink and its high Vitamin C content promotes collagen production, and it is effective in treating a wide range of stomach conditions from ulcers, acid, diarrhoea to constipation as well as having positive effects on gall stones, urinary tract infections and gout. The natural anti-inflammatory properties in rosehip tea make it good for arthritis, reducing pain and increasing mobility. It has also shown to be effective at reducing the symptoms of asthma, and helps to lower cholesterol and maintain healthy blood pressure levels, as well as regulating blood sugar levels, making it a useful tea for diabetics. As a natural diuretic and laxative, it aids the removal of toxins and waste from the body.

Interesting Fact – Did you know that rosehips played an important role in the provision of vitamin C to children during the Second World War, and that by 1945, more than 450 tonnes were harvested annually?

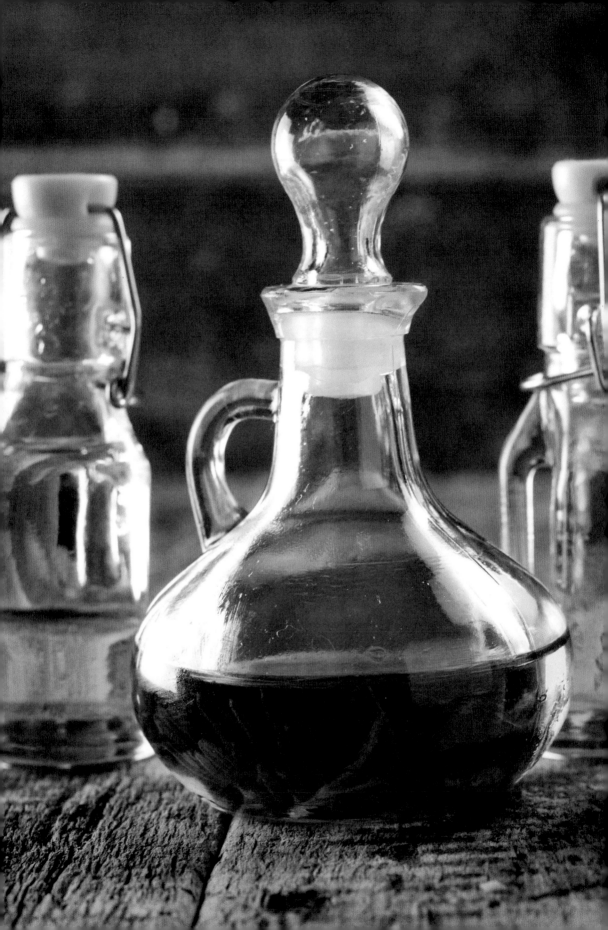

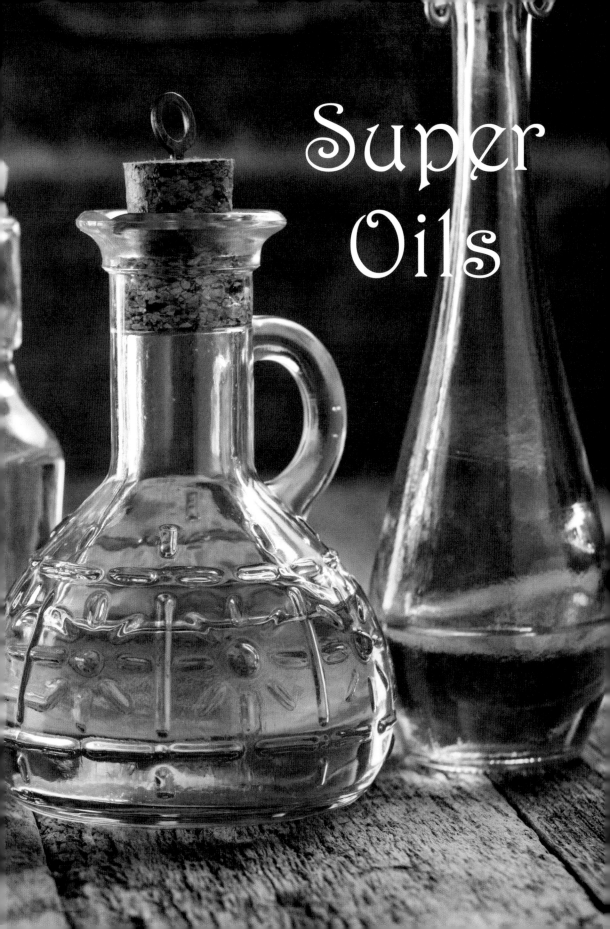

Super
Oils

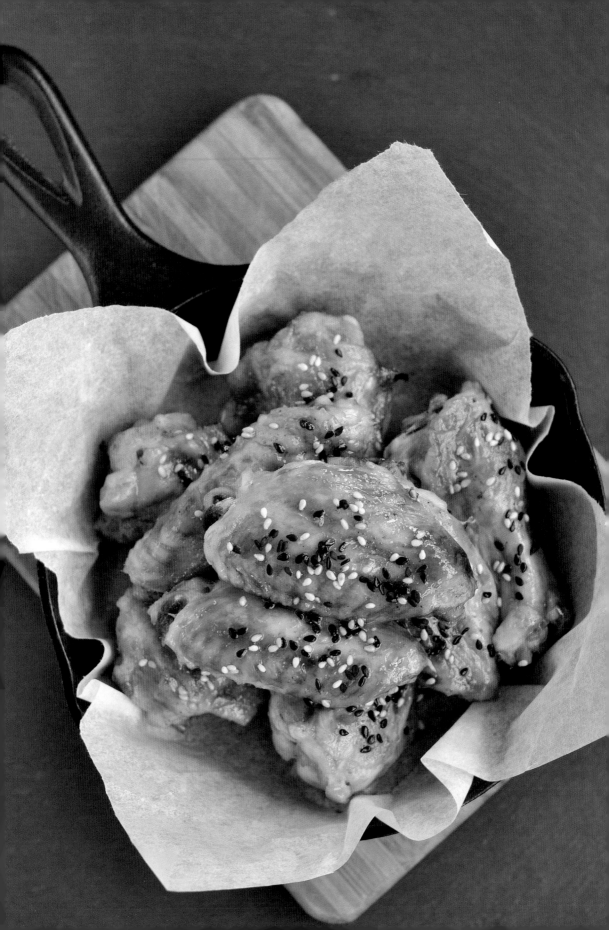

You only need to visit the supermarket now to realize what a huge selection of oils are readily available these days. There are oils from nuts, seeds, fruits and vegetables, all with different and distinct flavours and properties – and fabulous health benefits. I could easily have mentioned many of the oils detailed here in previous sections, but I feel that oils are of such importance that they deserve a category of their own. It also gives me the opportunity to explain not only the health benefits of each oil and the flavours they can bring to your dinner table, but also how best to use them. When cooking with oils, each oil handles heat differently – they each have their own 'smoke point'. This is the temperature at which the oil starts to break down, and once this happens, it loses it nutritional content and can very often assume an extremely bitter and rather unpleasant taste. The oil oxidizes which basically means it reacts with oxygen, forming harmful compounds which we do not want to consume.

But before we arrive at the cooking stage, please remember that all oils are extremely sensitive to both heat and light, which can also affect their nutrient content and flavour so always store in a cool, dark place and ensure you read the labels correctly as certain oils need to be refrigerated. If in doubt, a good test is to smell it and if it smells bitter or 'off' then throw it away. Some oils store for longer than others – polyunsaturated oils like grape seed oil or walnut oil tend to turn rancid more quickly. So which oils are super oils and how best should you utilize them?

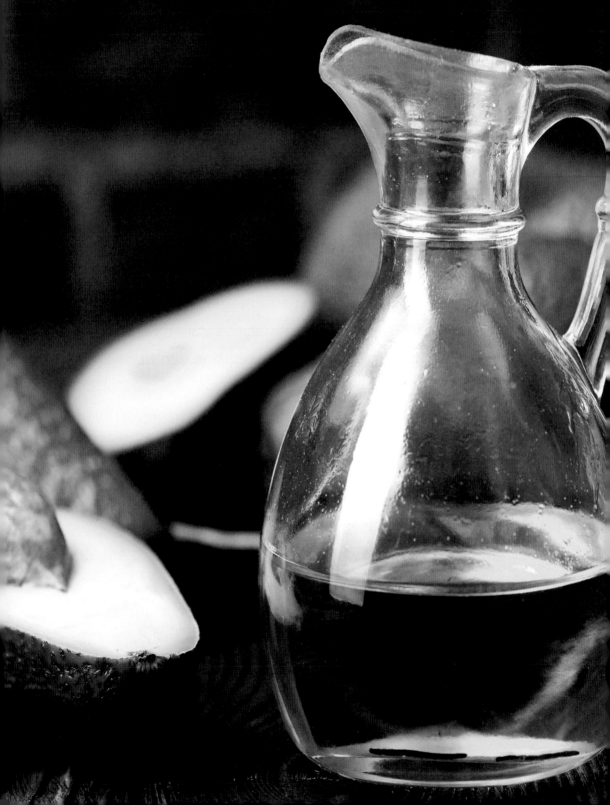

Avocado Oil

Avocado Oil Popcorn

This doesn't get any simpler. Simply pop your kernels as usual then toss in avocado oil (a little goes a long way so don't be too generous!) and enjoy! This is a prime example of nutritious yet still delicious.

Avocado oil is actually quite similar in composition to olive oil and therefore can be used for many of the same purposes. It is obtained from pressing the fleshy pulp of the avocado. It has a high smoke point so it works well with both grilling and frying. A good source of protein and vitamins A, D and E, it also contains beta carotene and lecithin. Extremely rich in monounsaturated oleic acid, which is known to prevent the absorption of cholesterol and prevent plaque formation. Studies have shown that consuming avocado oil on a regular basis significantly reduces the risk of thrombosis and heart disease. Good for the skin and high in anti-inflammatories, avocado oil also contains the anti-cancer properties, alpha linolenic acid and Omega-3 fatty acids. There have been four studies showing the positive results of avocado oil in reducing the symptoms of arthritis, and people who regularly consume avocado have been shown to have lower BMIs and less belly fat.

Uses – This oil will add a fantastic richness and flavour to your food. Try making avocado oil mayonnaise, or use it for the most wonderful salad and pasta dressings. Avocado hollandaise is delicious and the oil can be used in place of egg when dipping foods prior to coating in breadcrumbs or flour.

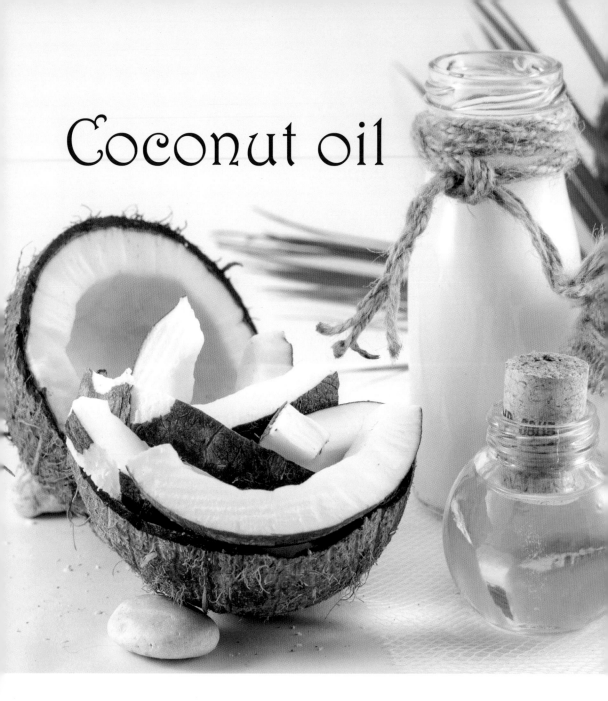

Coconut oil

I am sure you can't have missed the extraordinary rise in popularity of coconut oil in recent years. Often talked about in the press as a vital ingredient in many new health foods, the sales of coconut oil in the UK have tripled in the last year from £4.4 million to £13 million. At room temperature, coconut oil is solid, and it only transitions to liquid at between 24 and 26°C. More than 90 per cent of its fatty acids are saturated, making it the number one choice for cooking, as it maintains all its nutrients even when cooked at a high heat. It can also last for months and even years without going rancid.

However, coconut oil is special for many more reasons than its suitability for cooking. The saturated fat it contains are MCT's which are medium chain triglycerides – which

Coconut Oil Chocolate

Ingredients

½ cup of coconut oil
¼ cup of raw cacao powder
2 tablespoons of raw honey

1 teaspoon of vanilla extract
(optional)

Melt the coconut oil and add the honey. Start whisking, whilst adding he cacao powder and vanilla extract if using.

Once the ingredients are combined well, pour into ice cube trays and chill or freeze for 30 minutes until solid.

are fatty acids of medium length and these are metabolized differently to the long chain fatty acids. They go directly from the liver to the digestive tract making them an excellent quick source of energy, but they have also been shown to have therapeutic effects on brain disorders such as epilepsy or Alzheimer's disease. These MCT's have also been proven to increase calories burned as well as supressing the appetite, making coconut oil a popular choice for aiding weight loss. In fact, studies showed that the use of coconut oil in particular was effective at reducing belly fat.

Coconut oil is rich in lauric acid which can kill off bacteria and viruses and so helps to prevent infection and illness. It has also been shown to improve cholesterol, raising the levels of 'good' cholesterol and reducing the 'bad' cholesterol. Countries in which coconuts and their fats make up a large part of the diet have shown to be extremely healthy with little or no incidence of heart disease. Coconut oil also promotes a healthy thyroid and endocrine system, boosts liver, kidney and gallbladder health and facilitates the absorption of important minerals such as calcium and magnesium, helping to build strong bones and healthy teeth. I often use coconut oil on my hair which leaves it silky smooth but it is great too for the skin and aids healing when applied directly to wounds.

Uses – I could write a whole book on the uses of coconut oil. It is great for stir fries and I make a delicious chocolate spread by mixing coconut oil with raw cacao. Use it in the baking of cakes, breads, granolas, in muffins, to roast vegetables, or add to smoothies, lattes and hot chocolates. It is also great in sauces and dressings.

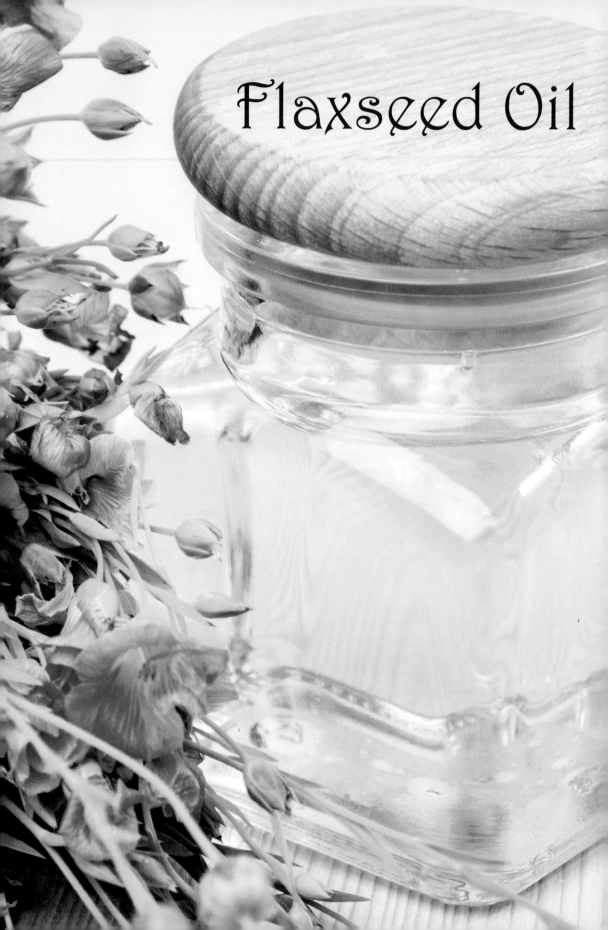

Flaxseed Oil

Quinoa and Chickpea Lettuce Wrap

I actually realized just how useful lettuce leaves can be for wraps after I was diagnosed as being allergic to gluten several years ago. At the time I was upset as it meant no more paninis on the go! However, after a little trial and error, I realized that living without gluten opened up a whole new world of flavours, products and recipes. Lettuce wraps were one of my success stories, not just for me, but for my whole family. We are always experimenting with different flavours and this one using flaxseed oil is particularly delicious.

Ingredients

Romain Lettuce Leaves
1 cup diced cucumber
1 cup grated carrots
½ cup cooked chick peas
1 cup shredded kale
2 cups cooked quinoa

1 cup diced red pepper
2 tablespoons flaxseed oil
2 tablespoons lemon juice
1 teaspoon Dijon mustard
Salt and pepper to taste

Mix the flaxseed oil, mustard, lemon juice and a little salt and pepper and whisk.

Add to the cucumber, grated carrots, chick peas, quinoa, kale and pepper and stir well. Load into the lettuce leaves – quick and simple.

Flaxseed oil or linseed oil, as it is also known, is the oil that is extracted from the dried ripe seeds of the flaxseed plant. This oil is becoming increasingly popular due to its high levels of Omega-3 and Omega-6 fatty acids which are heart healthy super powers, lowering cholesterol and preventing the build-up of plaque on the arteries. They are also useful for maintaining a healthy blood pressure. A fantastic natural anti-inflammatory, flaxseed oil may help improve conditions such as arthritis, gout and even asthma. With its high fibre content, it has been linked to improved intestine, bowel and digestive health, and for regulating hormones in women, thus reducing menopause symptoms and PMT as well as reducing potentially the risk of breast cancer. Flaxseed oil also promotes the growth of healthy nails, hair and skin. Flaxseed oil is not suitable for use at high temperatures but it can be added to pasta, mashed potatoes, soup or vegetables and I love it as a salad dressing.

Interesting Fact – A Harvard Study titled 'The preventable causes of death in the United States' revealed that between 72,000 and 96,000 deaths are caused annually due to an Omega-3 deficiency in the USA.

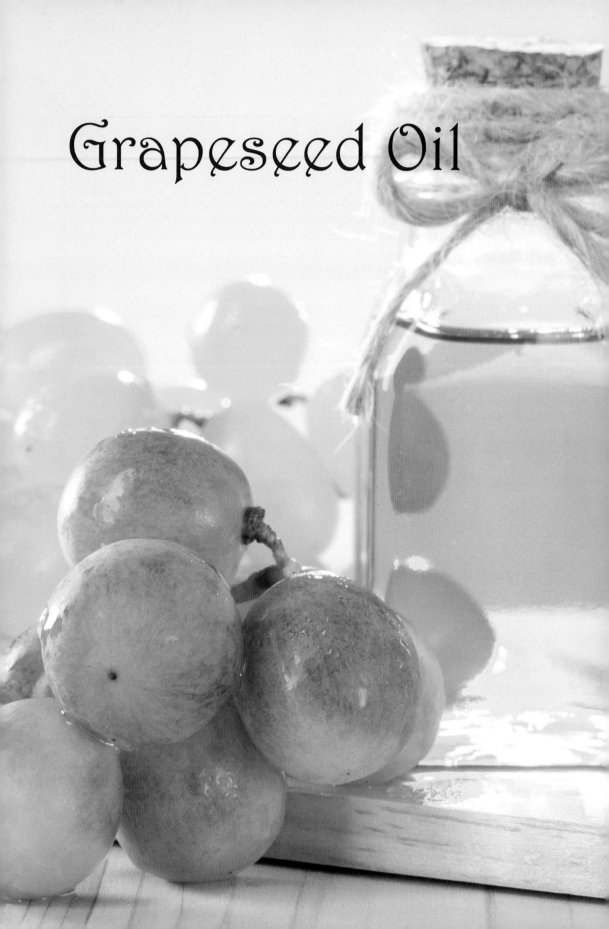

Grapeseed Oil

Golden Aubergines

Ingredients

An aubergine	2 egg whites
Salt	Grapeseed oil
Pepper	

Slice the aubergines and sprinkle with salt. Leave for 30 minutes (this process removes the bitterness). Rinse well, removing all the salt and pat dry. Season with salt and pepper.

Whisk the egg whites then brush each slice on both sides.

Heat several tablespoons of grapeseed oil in a wide bottom pan over a high heat and using no more than three to four slices at a time, place the aubergines into the pan and cook on both sides for around three minutes until golden and crisp.

Remove from the pan and place on a piece of kitchen towel. Continue with the process until all the slices have been cooked.

So we have already discussed the truly astounding health assets of grape seeds and there really could be no easier way of harnessing these benefits than by using grape seed oil. Light in colour and flavour with a hint of nuttiness. Best kept refrigerated, with a high smoke point so useful for cooking at high temperatures, it doesn't separate when used for making items such as mayonnaise. Rich in antioxidants and especially high in vitamin E, it also aids in the reduction of bad cholesterol. Useful for diabetics, it boosts circulation and the immune system. It is also a fantastic natural anti-inflammatory and so may reduce the symptoms of inflammatory conditions such as arthritis and asthma. The high Omega-6 content aids the body in burning fat and boosts energy. And don't just keep it for cooking, grape seed oil has shown to be an effective moisturizer in both beauty and haircare products. It sooths and nourishes the skin, tones, reduces wrinkles and stretch marks. It works fantastically as a base for salad dressings but can be used for baking, sautéing, stir frying and roasting.

Take note – If you are using cholesterol or blood pressure lowering drugs or blood thinning drugs, please consult your doctor before use.

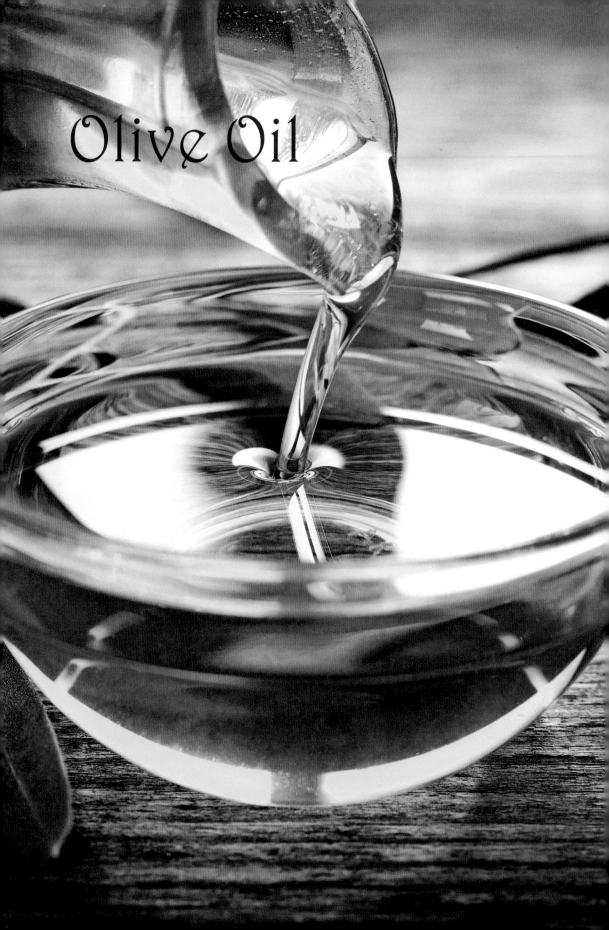

Olive Oil

Basil Pesto

Ingredients

3 tablespoons of pine nuts

3 cups basil leaves (no stems)

1 clove of garlic

½ cup of extra virgin olive oil

½ cup of freshly grated parmesan

Place all the ingredients in a food processor or blender except the parmesan and blend until smooth.

Add the cheese and mix only until combined. Fantastic served with pasta, meats or vegetables.

As mentioned earlier, I currently live in Spain and the Spanish use olive oil on and with everything. I have never sat at a table yet that doesn't have a bottle of olive oil on it or entered a kitchen that isn't adorned with a variety of bottles and brands of this delicious oil. Olive oil is a staple in some of the world's healthiest populations and is quite simply the oil that is obtained from pressing the olives that come from the olive tree. Always look for extra virgin olive oil that is the purest form and extracted using natural methods – there are other forms available of lesser quality that are often extracted using chemicals and on occasions, mixed with other cheaper oils, so choose carefully.

Containing good levels of vitamins, healthy fatty acids and absolutely bursting with antioxidants, olive oil is a fantastic natural anti-inflammatory, helps to lower both cholesterol and blood pressure and is thought to prevent blood clotting, making it a super heart healthy oil and good for preventating heart disease and strokes. Various studies have shown that those living in the Mediterranean countries are at lower risk for developing cancer and many believe this is due to the high consumption of olive oil. It is also thought to improve brain function.

Uses – My daughter absolutely loves soaking her bread in olive oil and we also add it to salads, pasta and vegetables. I often replace other fats in recipes for olive oil and try poaching tuna in it as it is just fabulous.

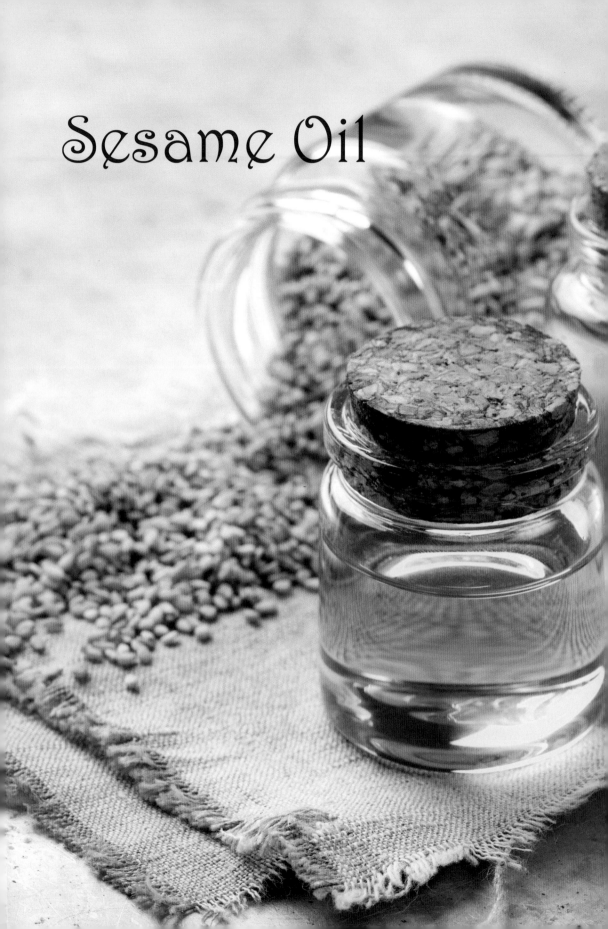

Sesame Oil

Sesame Oil Chicken Wings

Ingredients

2lbs chicken wings
¼ cup of sesame oil
1 cup of water

10 tablespoons of dark soy sauce
5 tablespoons of light soy sauce
1 green onion chopped

Place the chicken in a large cooking pot with the water, green onion and soy sauces and cook for 15 minutes on a medium heat.

Add the sesame oil and cook for a further 15 minutes until the chicken is cooked through and the sauce is sticky. Serve with rice and sprinkled with sesame seeds.

Sesame oil is one of the oldest extracted oils in history and once the most sought after oil in ancient India. Whilst sesame oil has been used for many years for a wide range of healing and medicinal purposes, recent studies and research have begun to confirm what our ancestors seemed to know long ago. The use of sesame oil regularly helps to reduce both blood pressure and sodium levels in the body as well as balancing blood sugar levels, and its anti-inflammatory and antibacterial strength help to prevent infection and reduce pain within the body.

A super skin food, sesame oil aids in the reduction of premature ageing as well as treating and preventing a wide range of skin conditions. A heart healthy oil, its high content of minerals such as magnesium, calcium, copper and zinc make it a bone booster too. It contains the feel good amino acid tyrosine, meaning it may also raise mood and reduce depression and anxiety. Sesame oil can also be used as nose drops to treat sinusitis, as a mouth wash or throat gargle, killing off infection and bacteria.

Uses – Sesame oil is particularly popular in Asian cuisine and inspired dishes. Salmon is wonderful marinated in soy and sesame sauce prior to roasting and peanut noodles are lovely with ginger, sesame oil and peanut butter. Try cooking green beans and broccoli in sesame oil and then sprinkling them with soy sauce and sesame seeds. Tuna is delicious cooked in sesame oil coated in sesame seeds.

Take note – If you are taking blood thinning medication please check with your doctor before adding sesame oil into your diet.

Walnut Oil

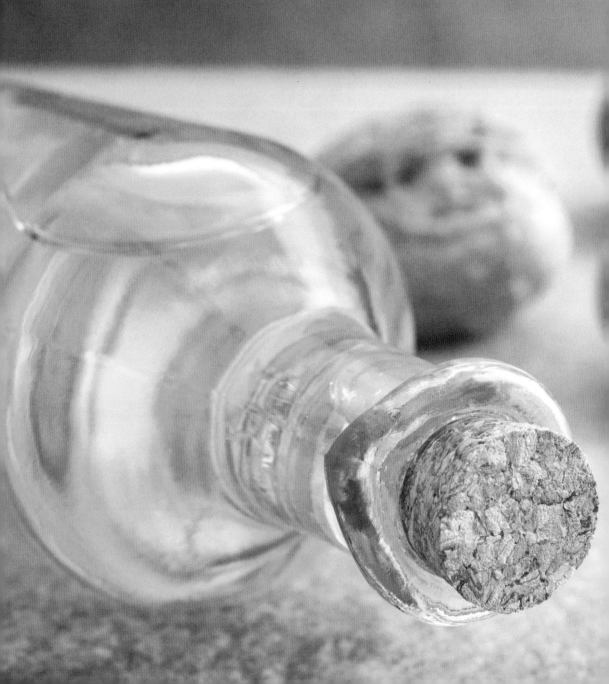

Walnut Oil Vinaigrette

Ingredients

¼ cup white wine vinegar
1 tablespoon minced shallot
2 teaspoons Dijon mustard
½ teaspoon salt

½ teaspoon ground black pepper
½ cup vegetable oil
¼ cup of walnut oil

Whisk together the vinegar, shallot, mustard, salt and pepper then add in a constant stream, whisking continuously the vegetable oil. Add the walnut oil and whisk further. This is amazing served over chargrilled asparagus and then topped with chopped walnuts.

Again we have already discussed the benefits of walnuts and this oil encapsulates all of these and is in a form that is so versatile and flavoursome. Not suitable for heating, as it will lose both its flavour and nutrient content, it is rich in heart healthy Omega-3 fatty acids which help to reduce cholesterol and prevent clotting. A fantastic natural anti-inflammatory, it is rich in antioxidants, especially vitamins C and E so boosting the immune system, collagen production, fighting the ageing process and the damage from harmful free radical and boosting healthy youthful skin. The monounsaturated fats help to control blood sugar levels and it contains the perfect balance of minerals to make it a bone boosting oil. Promoting brain health and aiding memory too. Use to drizzle over salads, cooked or raw vegetables, meats, and cheeses, pastas and soups.

Healthy Eating Tips

I thought to finish off I would just leave you with a few of my healthy hints to maximise your nutrient intake and provide the best environment for your body to absorb those nutrients.

1. **Try to prepare and cook your meals using fresh and organic ingredients.** Ready-made meals are high in salt and sugar as well as other additives and preservatives.
2. **Always read the nutrition label on your foods.** A good rule to follow is that if a food contains more than five ingredients, it probably isn't that good for you
3. **Eat five or more different coloured fruit and vegetables daily – seven if possible.** This will provide a wide range of nutrients. Raw juices and smoothies can count towards your daily intake too, and are actually an excellent way to get a powerhouse of vital vitamins and minerals into the body in an easily digestible form.
4. **Choose healthier cooking methods.** So bake, grill, steam, roast and stir fry
5. **Eat less red meat and more fish.** The health dangers of red meat have been highly documented with the most recent studies concluding that each bacon sandwich eaten takes an hour off your life expectancy! Fish is rich in protein, vitamins and minerals and oily fish is also high in essential omega fats.
6. **Choose healthy oils for cooking such as olive oil, grapeseed oil and coconut oil.** Grapeseed oil and coconut oil are excellent for maintaining all their nutrients even when cooked at high temperatures.
7. **Add little or no salt to your food.** Instead flavour your food with herbs and spices, pepper, garlic or lemon all of which are highly nutritious.
8. **Aim to drink at least eight to ten glasses of water daily.** I always have a bottle of water with me and drink continually throughout the day. Herbal teas and fruit juices also count.
9. **Buy organic –** Many people are unsure whether it is worth buying organic but my personal opinion is that it is. I am a huge fan of organic foods and believe they are worth the extra expense.
10. **Take time to enjoy your three meals a day.** Eat slowly, chew your food properly and do not eat whilst sat at your desk, watching TV or on the computer as this distracts you from the amount of food you are eating and can lead to overeating.

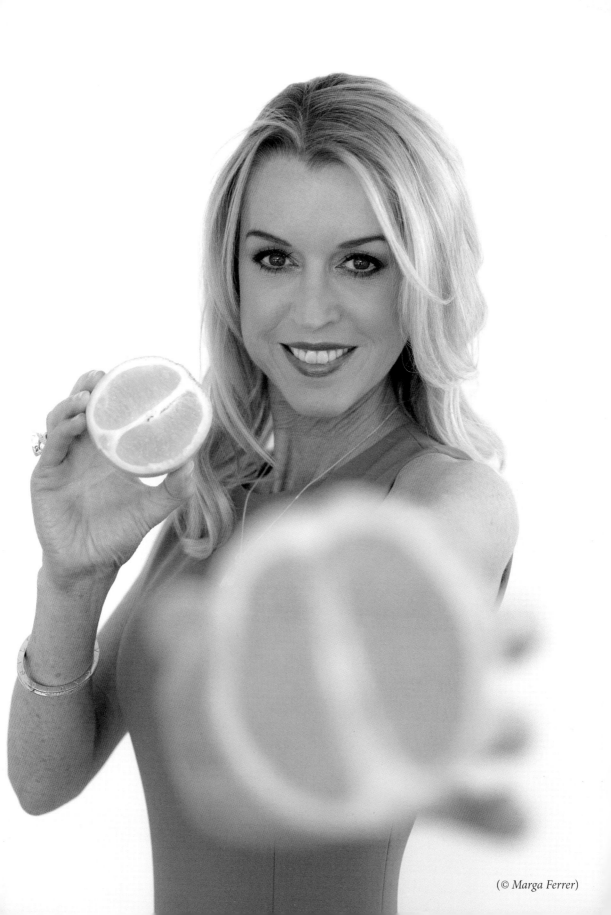

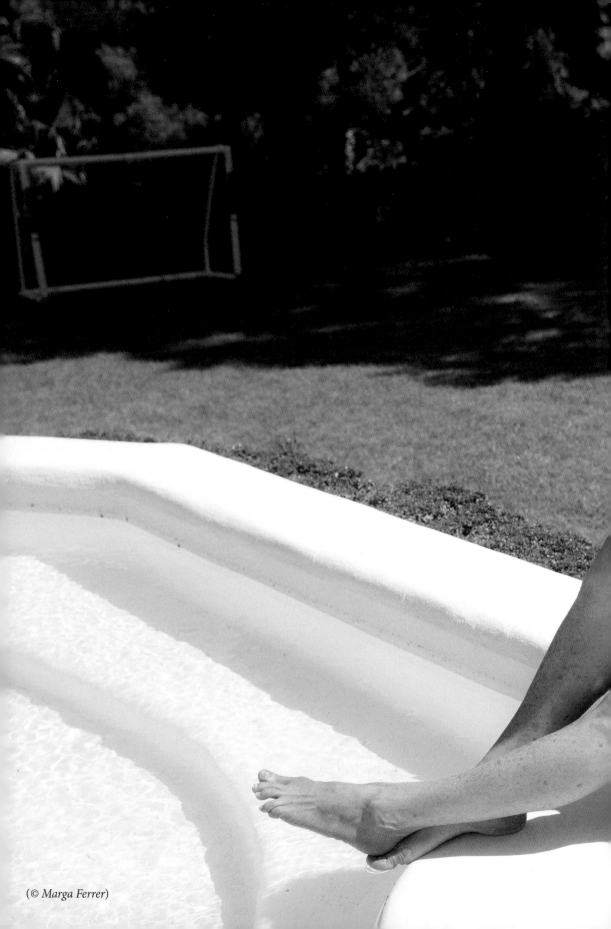

(© Marga Ferrer)

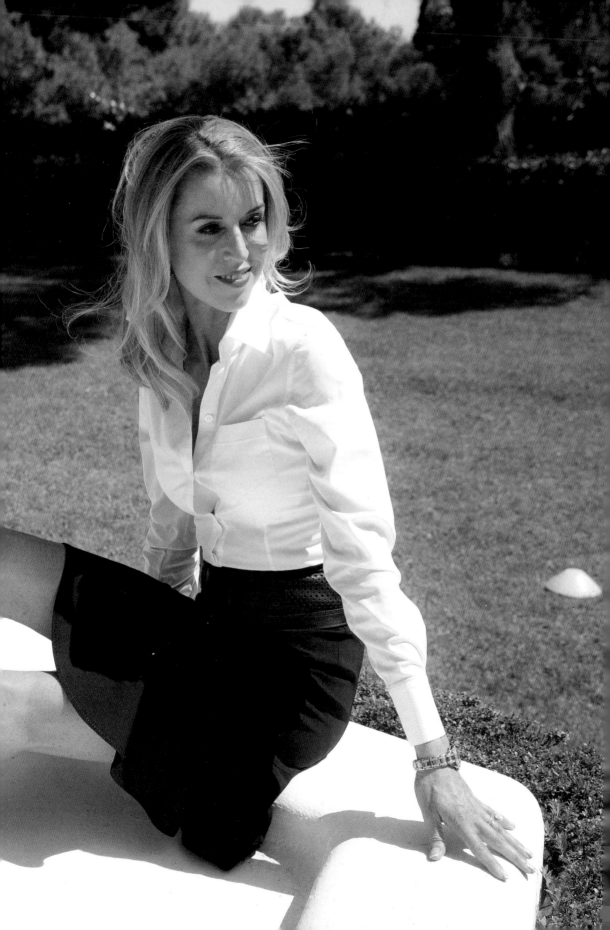

Measurements

As there are a wide range of recipes included in this book, I thought it would be useful to include the measurement conversions as everyone seems to have their favourites they like to work with.

NOTE: THESE ALL NEED TO BE CHECKED VERY CAREFULLY

Spoons:

British	American
1 teaspoon	1 teaspoon
1 tablespoon	1 tablespoon
2 tablespoons	3 tablespoons
3.5 tablespoons	4 tablespoons
4 tablespoons	5 tablespoons

Solid measures:
Using the one cup standard measure as sold here in the UK (NB: Please remember to alter the amount for your own recipe)

British	American
1lb (450g) butter or margarine	2 cups (or four sticks)
1lb (450g) flour	4 cups
1lb (450g) granulated or caster (superfine), sugar	2 cups
1lb (450g) icing sugar (confectioners' sugar)	3 cups
4oz (110g) icing sugar (confectioner's sugar)	½ cup plus a heaped tablespoon
8oz (225g) flour	2 cups
110g flour	1 cup

British	American
225g breadcrumbs	2 cups
110g breadcrumbs	1 cup
225g oatmeal	2 cups
4oz (110g) oatmeal	1 cup
8oz (225g) grated cheese	2 cups
4oz (110 g) grated cheese	1 cup.
8oz (225g) butter, margarine, or shortening	1 cup (or 2 sticks)
4oz (110g) butter, margarine, or shortening	1/2 cup (or 1 stick)
2oz (50g) butter, margarine or shortening	¼ cup (1/2 a stick)
4oz (110g) dried mixed fruit, (fruitcake mix)	2/3 cup
2oz (50g) dried mixed fruit, (fruit cake mix)	1/3 cup
8oz (225g) brown sugar	1 cup
4oz (110g) brown sugar	½ cup
3oz (75g) chocolate, broken into squares	¾ cup
4oz (110g) whole hazelnuts	1 cup
2oz (50g) flaked, (slivered) almonds	½ cup
4 oz, 110 g, ground almonds	1 cup

Teaspoon measures:

1oz (25g), is one heaped teaspoon of flour, oatmeal, cheese, breadcrumbs, or icing, confectioner's grade sugar.

1oz (25g), is 1 rounded teaspoon of granulated or caster, superfine, sugar.

1oz, (25g), is 2 level tbsp of butter, margarine or shortening.

Liquid measures:

British	American
Half teaspoon (2.5ml)	teaspoon
2.5 ml, 1 tsp, 5 ml	1 teaspoon
5 ml	1 average tablespoon
15 ml	1 average teaspoon
15 ml	A quarter of a pint
150 ml	Two thirds of a cup
120ml, 4 fl.oz	half a cup
½ pint	275ml
8 fl.oz	A genenerous cup
¾ pint, 425 ml.	2 cups
1 pint (570ml)	2½ cups
1½ pints (840 ml)	3¾ cups
1¾ pints (1 litre)	4½ cups
2 pints	5 cups

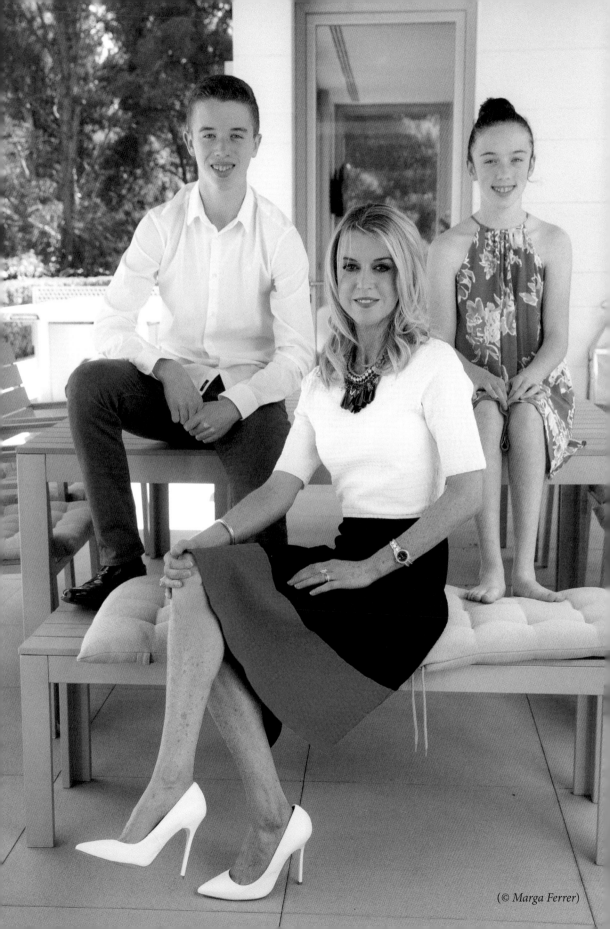

(© Marga Ferrer)

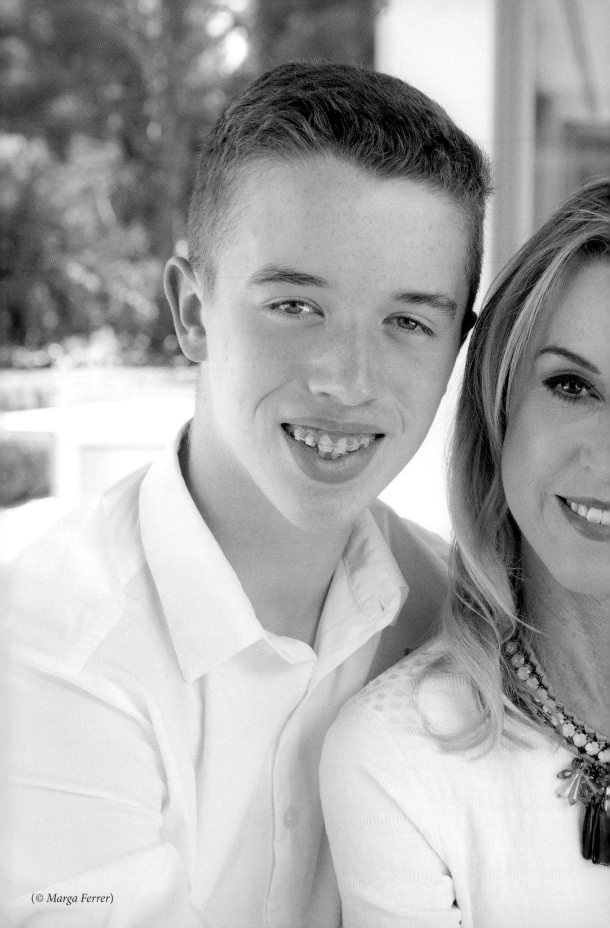

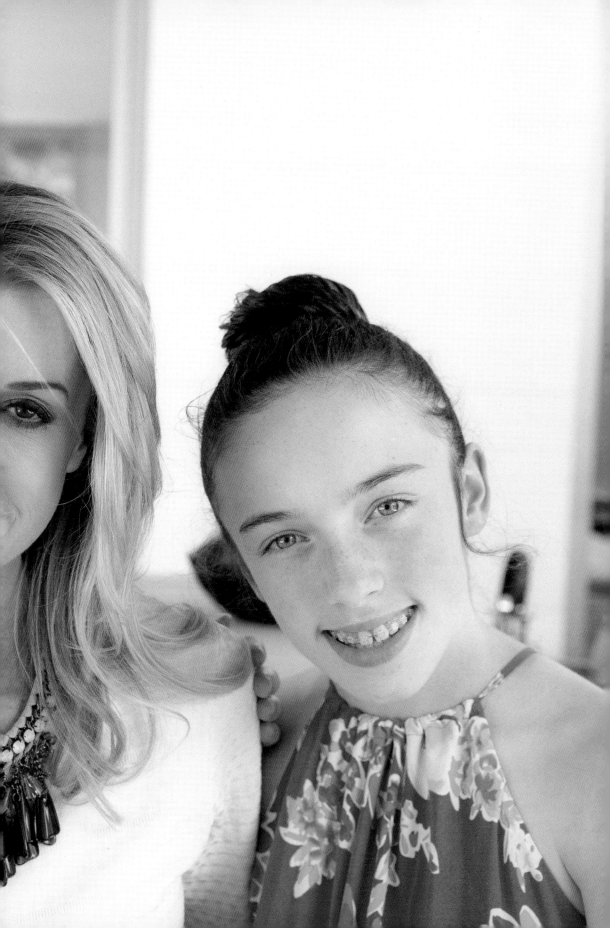

Index